Therapeutics and Pharmacology
for medical students

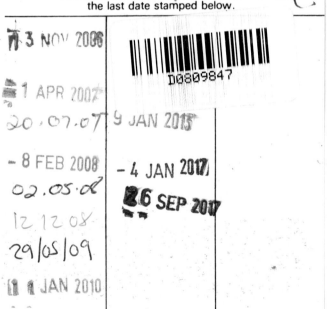

This book is to be returned on or before
the last date stamped below.

PasTest

Therapeutics and Pharmacology
for medical students

Paul Hamilton BSc (Hons) MRCP (UK)
Specialist Registrar in Clinical Pharmacology
Belfast City Hospital, Belfast

David McCluskey MD (Hons), FRCP (Lon)
FRCP (Edin) FRCPI
Consultant Physician
Royal Victoria Hospital, Belfast and
Head of Division of Medicine and Therapeutics
Queen's University of Belfast, Belfast

Dennis Johnston DSc MD PhD FRCP FRCPI
Consultant Physician
Belfast City Hospital, Belfast and
Professor of Medicine and Therapeutics,
Queen's University of Belfast, Belfast

Dr Catherine Ritchie MD, FRCP, MPhil
Consultant Physician
Craigavon Area Hospital, Craigavon

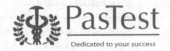

PasTest

Dedicated to your success

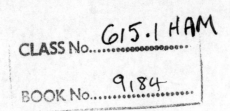
First edition 2006

ISBN: 1 904627 67 6
ISBN: 978 1 904627 67 8

A catalogue record for this book is available from the British Library.

The information contained within this book was obtained by the authors from reliable sources. However, while every effort has been made to ensure its accuracy, no responsibility for loss, damage or injury occasioned to any person acting or refraining from action as a result of information contained herein can be accepted by the publishers or author.

Every effort has been made to contact holders of copyright to obtain permission to reproduce copyright material at the time of going to press. However, if any have been inadvertently overlooked, the publisher will be pleased to make the necessary arrangements at the first opportunity.

PasTest Revision Books and Intensive Courses

PasTest has been established in the field of postgraduate medical education since 1972, providing revision books and intensive study courses for doctors preparing for their professional examinations.

Books and courses are available for the following specialties:

MRCGP, MRCP Parts 1 and 2, MRCPCH Parts 1 and 2, MRCPsych, MRCS, MRCOG Parts 1 and 2, DRCOG, DCH, FRCA, PLAB Parts 1 and 2.

For further details contact:

PasTest, Freepost, Knutsford, Cheshire WA16 7BR

Tel: 01565 752000   **Fax: 01565 650264**

www.pastest.co.uk   **enquires@pastest.co.uk**

Text prepared by Carnegie Book Production, Lancaster
Printed by MPG Books Ltd, Bodmin, Cornwall

Contents

Acknowledgements

For my grandparents

PH

Introduction

The aim of this book is to provide medical students with a concise yet comprehensive overview of therapeutics and pharmacology that is pitched at the right level and covers all the information required. It is by no means a reference text, but has been written with the busy medical student in mind. It covers all areas that would be expected in most medical school curricula.

The chapters have been written in a manner that reflects clinical practice. We have concentrated on commonly prescribed drugs, rather than aiming to detail every medication on the market. Students who have read and understood this book will be in an excellent position to excel in undergraduate examinations, and will find drug prescribing a rewarding and exciting challenge as they enter their foundation years in clinical medicine.

Chapters 1 and 2 outline the scientific principles that underlie drug development and use. This is followed by systems-based chapters, which form the main body of the book. Within each system, the commonly prescribed classes of drugs are described. For most drugs, the following system has been used to facilitate learning:

- Mechanism of action: how the drug works.
- Examples: a non-exhaustive list, which should help you answer questions such as 'Name a few β blockers'.
- Example prescription: this provides an example 'real prescription' to give you a feel for how you might 'write up' a drug. The doses illustrated are just typical examples, and are not correct in all settings. Box 1 details elements of good prescribing that are used throughout the book.
- Indications: these are listed when not immediately obvious.
- Contraindications: important contraindications are listed. These are not exhaustive, but are the most commonly occurring contraindications in day-to-day practice. Most drugs have relative contraindications for their use, and these should always be checked in the product literature or the *British National Formulary* (BNF) when prescribing a drug.
- Common side effects: drugs often have many side effects associated with them. To facilitate learning, only those that occur commonly are listed in this book.

- Significant interactions: again, multiple drug interactions are recognised. Appendix 1 in the BNF lists these interactions in detail. It would be very difficult for anyone to remember all these interactions, especially as the clinically relevant ones are relatively few in number. We have highlighted the common and most dangerous drug interactions here and, when it has been stated that there are no interactions, this relates to common occurrences. You are encouraged to check carefully for potential drug interactions each and every time you prescribe a drug.

Box 1 Good prescribing

A standard prescription is written in the following order:

Name of drug, dose, route of delivery and frequency of delivery.

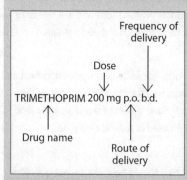

Figure 1 Example of a drug prescription.

As far as possible, prescribe drugs using their generic names. Avoid using proprietary names (names used by drugs companies) unless absolutely neccessary. For example, document Omeprazole rather than Losec®. Those preparations that include more than one drug or that are special formulations (such as slow release) may need the proprietary name to be noted. For example, Adalat® SR is acceptable for the slow release preparation of nifedipine.

- Always print drug names in capital letters. This helps nurses and others decipher handwriting more easily.

- Always write doses clearly, adhering to the following rules:

    Use the most appropriate units, eg 10 000 micrograms would be better written as 10 mg

    Never use a 'trailing zero', because 10.0 g could easily be misinterpreted as 100 g. The correct prescription would state 10 g.

    Do not use abbreviations for non-standard units.

    Grams may be shortened to g.

Box 1 Good prescribing *(continued)*

Milligrams may be shortened to mg.

Micrograms should never be shortened, ie write the full word.

Nanograms should never be shortened, ie write the full word.

Picograms should never be shortened, ie write the full word.

Units should never be shortened, ie write the full word.

- Abbreviations can be used for common routes of drug delivery as shown here:

  p.o. = oral

  i.v. = intravenous

  i.m. = intramuscular

  s.c. = subcutaneous

  s.l. = sublingual

  p.r. = rectal.

- The frequency of drug delivery can also be abbreviated as shown:

  o.d. = *omni die* = once daily

  b.d. = *bis die* = twice daily

  t.i.d. = *ter in die* = three times daily

  q.i.d. = *quater in die* = four times daily

  p.r.n. = *pro re nata* = when required (always specify a minimum time interval between doses and a maximum daily dose)

  stat = immediately

  mane = in the morning

  nocte = at night.

We would encourage you to use this book as a companion to your medical studies. It will help you in with preclinical work and be a good guide as you progress through clinical attachments.

1
Principles of pharmacology

1
Principles of pharmacology

Pharmacology is the study of the effects of specific chemical entities (drugs or medications) on processes within the body, whereas therapeutics is defined as the use of drugs in the treatment of disease. To produce a therapeutic effect a drug must achieve sufficient concentration at its site of action. The processes involved in achieving adequate amounts of drug within the body are referred to as 'pharmacokinetics', whereas the term 'pharmacodynamics' is used to describe the mode of action. In other words, pharmacokinetics describes what the body does to a drug, whereas pharmacodynamics refers to what a drug does to the body.

Absorption, distribution, metabolism and excretion all involve movement across cell membranes. The nature of cell membranes and the physiochemical properties of drug molecules will influence the concentrations in different parts of the body.

The cell membrane

A large proportion of mammalian cell membranes consists of a double layer of phospholipid molecules arranged so that their hydrophilic heads are situated at the inner and outer surfaces of the membrane while their hydrophobic segments occupy the central core (Figure 1.1). Proteins are also present in the plasma membrane and consist of two forms – intrinsic and extrinsic. Intrinsic proteins span the lipid bilayer and include transporter molecules and receptors for hormones and neurotransmitters. Extrinsic proteins are attached to either an intrinsic protein on the inner surface of the membrane or to hydrophilic phospholipid head groups at the external or internal surfaces. The cell membrane is a fluid structure in which the various components are mobile.

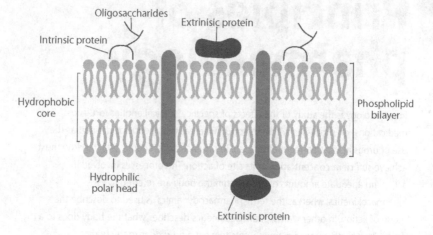

Figure 1.1 Schematic diagram of the cell membrane.

The movement of drugs across the cell membranes

There are four routes by which drugs cross cell membranes:

1. Passive diffusion through the phospholipid layer
2. Diffusion through aqueous pores in the membrane
3. Diffusion through intracellular pores
4. Carrier-mediated transport.

Passive diffusion through the phospholipid layer

Most drugs pass through cell membranes by simple passive diffusion down the concentration gradient. The rate of passive diffusion of a drug is related to its lipid solubility and the factors included in Fick's law of diffusion – the concentration gradient and the surface area and thickness of the membrane.

Fick's law of diffusion

This states that the rate of diffusion will be greatest when:

- The concentration on one side of a membrane is high
- The area over which diffusion can take place is large
- The membrane is thin.

This is represented by the following formula

$$\text{Rate of diffusion} = \frac{\text{Concentration gradient} \times \text{Permeability coefficient} \times \text{Area}}{\text{Thickness}}$$

Diffusion through pores (aqueous diffusion)

This is a passive process in which molecules move through small water-filled pores. The membranes of small capillaries permit the aqueous diffusion of molecules up to the size of small proteins between the blood and extravascular space.

Diffusion through intercellular pores

Some drugs (eg insulin) are large proteins and are unable to diffuse passively across cell membranes. However, these molecules can move across membranes by diffusing through the intercellular pores (50-100 μm in diameter). This is known as 'paracellular diffusion'.

Carrier-mediated transport

Active transport across cell membranes is achieved by two main processes.

Transport by special carriers

Drugs can be transported across barriers by mechanisms similar to those used to transfer endogenous substances, eg amino acid carriers in the blood–brain barrier and weak acid carriers in the renal tubule. Selective inhibition of these carriers can be used clinically to reduce urinary drug excretion, eg probenecid can reduce penicillin secretion by the renal tubule and weak acids can be used to reduce uric acid reabsorption.

Endocytosis and exocytosis

In these processes, drugs bind to specialised components on the cell membrane and produce infolding and internalisation of that area of the membrane. The contents of the resulting vesicle are then released into the cytoplasm. Large molecules such as peptides or smaller molecules combined with special proteins (eg vitamin B_{12} with intrinsic factor and iron with transferrin) can enter the cell by this mechanism.

Water and lipid solubility

The lipid solubility of a drug can be determined by measuring its distribution between an immiscible organic solvent and water – the oil:water partition coefficient.

The higher the partition coefficient, the greater the lipid solubility and the more rapidly the drug will diffuse across lipid cell membranes.

Overall, lipid-soluble molecules tend to be better absorbed after oral administration, distribute more widely within the body, are more subject to metabolism and less effectively excreted by the kidney.

For drugs that are weak bases or weak acids, the pH of the medium determines the ionised and unionised fractions of the molecule. If the pK_a (the pH at which 50% of the drug is ionised) and the pH of the medium are known, the fraction of the molecule in the ionised form can be calculated using the Henderson–Hasselbalch equation:

$$\log (\text{Protonated form/Unprotonated form}) = pK_a - pH$$

Weak bases are more polar and more water soluble when they are protonated, whereas weak acids are less water soluble when they are protonated. When a patient takes an overdose of a weak acidic drug, eg aspirin, its excretion can be accelerated by making the urine more alkaline. When the urinary pH is increased the weak acid dissociates to its charged, polar form and less diffuses from the renal tubule into the blood (Figure 1.2).

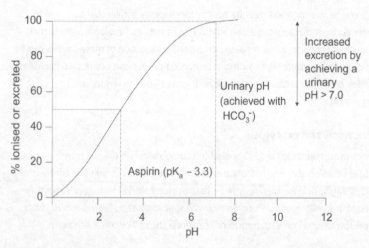

Figure 1.2 Relationship between urinary pH and the percentage of aspirin in the ionised or readily excreted form.

Drug absorption and distribution

Absorption

The absorption of a drug is defined as the movement of the drug from its site of administration into the plasma, from where it is distributed through the body. The routes of administration can be divided into two principal groups:

1. Enteral: oral, sublingual and rectal
2. Parenteral: intravenous, intramuscular, subcutaneous, inhalation and topical.

Enteral

Oral

This is the most popular route because of convenience. Absorption is slower and less complete compared to other forms of administration, and some drugs are subject to extensive first-pass metabolism in the liver or gut wall before they reach the systemic circulation. Some drugs, eg glyceryl trinitrate (GTN), have very low bioavailability when given orally because of extensive first-pass metabolism.

Buccal and sublingual

A method that is suitable for a small selection of drugs that are highly lipid soluble, eg organic nitrates. Sublingual or buccal GTN produces an immediate effect and avoids first-pass metabolism.

Rectal

This may be a useful route for some drugs to avoid local gastrointestinal irritation and first-pass metabolism. Local rectal irritation may occur, eg with non-steroidal anti-inflammatory drugs (NSAIDs).

Parenteral

Intravenous

Intravenous administration offers immediate and complete absorption but the risk of serious adverse events and acute allergic reactions (caused by high peak concentrations) is increased.

Intramuscular

In general, this method should be avoided. Although many drugs achieve higher concentrations at the site of action than after oral administration, a number of drugs, eg digoxin and phenytoin, are poorly absorbed, and can cause muscle necrosis or pain at the site of injection.

Subcutaneous

Absorption is usually slower than the intramuscular route and the volume of drug that can be given is limited. It is the route of first choice for insulin and heparin.

Inhalation

In respiratory disease this allows delivery to the target tissues and reduces systemic adverse effects. The rapid onset and offset of anaesthesia is often achieved by this route.

Topical

Application to skin and mucous membranes for local effect is widely used within medicine, eg for delivery to the eye, nose, throat or vagina. Systemic absorption is usually slower than with most other methods of drug administration.

Distribution

Following absorption into the plasma, a drug is available for distribution to interstitial and cellular fluids. The capillaries, with the exception of those in the brain and placenta, have endothelial membranes with intracellular pores that allow drugs to diffuse rapidly out of the vascular system. The movement of drugs into cells depends on the same factors that determine absorption from the gut – lipid solubility, molecular size and polarity. Other factors that influence the rate of distribution include the size of the organ in which distribution occurs, its associated blood flow and the degree of protein binding.

Size of the organ

Although the concentration in muscle may be relatively low, this tissue often acts as an important drug reservoir because of its very large mass of tissue. In contrast, similar amounts of drug will raise the concentrations more in the brain because of its relatively small size.

Blood flow

This is a major determinant of the rate of drug uptake by an organ but has limited impact on tissue steady-state concentrations. Well-perfused organs – brain, heart, kidneys and gut – will achieve higher concentrations earlier than poorly perfused tissues such as fat or bone.

Solubility

Lipid-soluble drugs distribute widely into tissues with a high lipid content. Most centrally acting drugs, including anaesthetics, are very lipid soluble and distribute into the brain more rapidly than water-soluble drugs.

Binding

Binding of a drug to macromolecules in the blood or tissues increases the amount within that compartment and reduces the amount in other compartments. Drugs that are extensively bound to plasma albumin, eg warfarin, tend to remain within the vascular compartment. Those drugs that have extensive tissue binding, eg digoxin, digitoxin, amiodarone and chloroquine, have low plasma concentrations and large apparent volumes of distribution.

The blood–brain barrier

The central nervous system (CNS) is surrounded by a specialised barrier that prevents the penetration of hydrophilic substances. Unlike capillaries in most other tissues, endothelial cells in the brain do not possess intracellular pores and are described as having tight junctions. In addition, glial cells within the brain substance provide a further barrier to the diffusion of hydrophilic drugs. Drugs therefore must be lipid soluble to diffuse rapidly into the brain.

Role of the placenta

The placenta performs an important role in separating the fetal from the maternal circulation and regulates the exchange of a number of substances between the two circulations. Overall, the placenta acts as a large lipid membrane so that ionised lipid-soluble drugs pass more easily than hydrophilic drugs.

Elimination

Drugs are eliminated from the body by a combination of metabolism and excretion. The main route of drug excretion is the kidney. Other routes include biliary, pulmonary, sweat and saliva.

Renal excretion

Renal excretion of drugs involves three basic processes:

1. Glomerular filtration
2. Active tubular secretion
3. Passive tubular reabsorption.

Glomerular filtration

Most drugs are small molecules (< 70 kDa) and undergo significant glomerular filtration. Polar, water-soluble molecules are filtered more easily but, when bound to albumin and other plasma proteins, they do not undergo filtration because of their molecular size. Highly protein-bound drugs, eg warfarin, therefore undergo little glomerular filtration.

Active secretion

Active secretion of organic acids (eg benzylpenicillin) and bases (eg pethidine) from the plasma takes place in the proximal tubule. This occurs against the concentration gradient and involves the transportation of protein-bound and -unbound drug. Competition for the carriers can occur which will reduce renal excretion. Probenecid (an organic acid) competitively inhibits the secretion of other organic acids, eg benzylpenicillin. This was used in the past to reduce the dose of benzylpenicillin required when it was in short supply.

Reabsorption

Most drugs undergo reabsorption. Lipid-soluble drugs will be reabsorbed along the whole length of the tubule. Weak acids and bases are not reabsorbed in their ionised form. The excretion of drugs by the kidney can therefore be altered by changing the urinary pH as previously described.

Drug excretion in patients with renal impairment

Patients with renal impairment, as a result of disease or age, will demonstrate reduced renal excretion of drugs that are primarily eliminated by this route. In clinical practice, creatinine clearance or serum creatinine is used to assess renal function and the ability of the kidney to excrete drugs. A number of nomograms using age, sex, serum creatinine and body mass are available for drugs that have a narrow therapeutic index and are eliminated by the kidney, eg aminoglycoside antibiotics. The lower the glomerular filtration rate, as assessed by creatinine clearance or serum creatinine, the lower the dose required for therapeutic effect. This can be achieved by reducing the individual doses and/or lengthening the dosing interval.

Biliary excretion

Drugs and their metabolites can be removed by excretion into the bile. Biliary excretion is an active process and occurs via transport systems for organic ions and neutral substances. Larger molecules (> 300 kDa) are more readily excreted. Drug conjugation, particularly glucuronidation, results in larger molecules being formed; these are more readily excreted. Also because they are more polar substances that are more poorly absorbed by the gastrointestinal tract after biliary excretion. Reabsorption can occur, however, with drugs that are highly lipid soluble or deconjugated in the gut to render them less polar. Glucuronides are deconjugated by the enzyme β1-glucuronidase. Biliary excretion and gut reabsorption can occur on a number of occasions. This process is known as 'enterohepatic recirculation'.

Metabolism of drugs

Drug metabolism involves the alteration of the chemical structure of a drug to create a more polar entity, which is then excreted by the kidney. For most drugs, metabolism takes place in the liver, catalysed by microsomal and sometimes non-microsomal enzymes. Drug-metabolising enzymes are also found in the lung, kidney, gastrointestinal tract and placenta. It is customary to divide the process of drug metabolism into phase I and phase II reactions.

Phase I reactions include oxidation (especially by the cytochrome P450 group of enzymes – mixed function oxidases), reduction, deamination and hydrolysis. Examples are included in Table 1.1.

Nature of the reaction	Common drug substrates
Oxidation: cytochrome P450-dependent	
Hydroxylation	Barbiturates, amfetamines, phenytoin
N-Dealkylation	Morphine, caffeine, theophylline
O-Dealkylation	Codeine
N-Oxidation	Paracetamol
S-Oxidation	Cimetidine, chlorpromazine
Deamination	Diazepam
Oxidation: cytochrome P450-independent	
Amine oxidation	Adrenaline (epinephrine)
Dehydrogenation	Ethanol
Reduction	Chloramphenicol, naloxone
Hydrolysis:	
Esters	Aspirin, suxamethonium
Amides	Procainamide, indometacin

Table 1.1 Phase I reactions

Phase II reactions are synthetic reactions involving the addition (conjugation) of subgroups to $-OH$, $-NH_2$ and $-SH$ radicals on the drug molecule. The subgroups added are glucuronate, acetate, glutathione, glycine, sulphate and methyl groups. Most are polar and make the molecule less lipid soluble. Examples are given in Table 1.2.

Nature of the reaction	Common drug substrates
Glucuronidation	Paracetamol, morphine, diazepam, digoxin
Acetylation	Isoniazid, clonazepam, sulphonamides
Glutathione conjugation	Paracetamol (oxidised metabolite)
Glycine conjugation	Aspirin, nicotinic acid
Sulphate conjugation	Paracetamol, methyldopa
Methylation	Catecholamines

Table 1.2 Phase II reactions

Factors that determine the rate of drug metabolism

Variation in the rate of metabolism between individuals is a result of genetic factors or interaction with other drugs. For a small number of drugs, age and disease have a significant effect, and gender has an effect on alcohol metabolism. Smoking is known to increase the metabolism of theophylline.

Genetic factors

There are three well-defined examples of variations in drug metabolism that are genetically determined: acetylation of amines, hydrolysis of esters and oxidation.

Acetylation of amines

A number of drugs are inactivated by N-acetylation. Individuals with deficient acetylation capacity, called 'slow acetylators', demonstrate increased plasma concentrations and adverse effects to drugs that undergo acetylation, eg isoniazid and procainamide (Figure 1.3). The percentages of slow acetylators varies between different populations (50% USA, 10-20% Japan). The slow acetylation trait is inherited as an autosomal recessive gene.

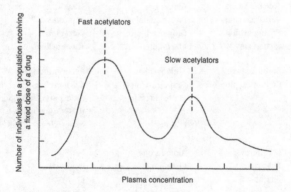

Figure 1.3 Distribution of plasma concentrations of drugs that are metabolised by acetylation, showing a clear bimodal distribution and the division into fast and slow acetylators.

Hydrolysis of esters

Approximately 1 in 2500 individuals has an abnormal form of the enzyme plasma cholinesterase. Suxamethonium is a muscle relaxant that is metabolised by plasma cholinesterase. The variant enzyme inactivates suxamethonium more slowly and can result in prolonged neuromuscular paralysis lasting several hours.

THERAPEUTICS AND PHARMACOLOGY FOR MEDICAL STUDENTS

Oxidation

The rate of oxidation of phenformin, metoprolol and some tricyclic antidepressants is genetically determined. Fast oxidisers show reduced pharmacological effect, whereas slow oxidisers are at increased risk of developing adverse effects.

Drug interactions

Enzyme induction

A large number of drugs increase the synthesis of cytochrome P450-dependent, drug-oxidising enzymes in the liver. Common inducers are listed in Table 1.3. Several days are usually required to reach maximum induction or to regress after withdrawal of the inducer. Some drugs induce their own metabolism. The overall effect is to reduce the pharmacological activity of the parent drug that undergoes oxidative metabolism.

CYP family	Inducers	Inhibitors	Drug with metabolism affected
1A2	Tobacco smoke Carbamazepine Phenobarbital Rifampicin	Cimetidine Fluoroquinolones Grapefruit juice Macrolides	Tricyclic antidepressants Paracetamol Clozapine Theophylline
3A4	Barbiturates Carbamazepine	Amiodarone Grapefruit juice Metronidazole	Azole antifungals Calcium channel blockers Ciclosporin, oestrogens HMG-CoA inhibitors, rifampicin
2C9	Barbiturates Phenytoin Rifampicin	Amiodarone Cimetidine Isoniazid Metronidazole SSRIs	Barbiturates Ibuprofen Phenytoin Chlorpromazine Warfarin
2C19	Carbamazepine Phenobarbital Phenytoin	Omeprazole SSRIs	Phenytoin Tricyclic antidepressants Warfarin

HMG-CoA, hydroxymethylglutaryl-coenzyme A; SSRIs, selective serotonin reuptake inhibitors.

Table 1.3 Examples of drugs that significantly induce or inhibit cytochrome P450 metabolism in humans and the drugs that are commonly affected

Enzyme inhibition

Common enzyme inhibitors are listed in Table 1.3. Unlike the process of enzyme induction, the process is usually rapid.

Drug-induced changes in liver blood flow

Decreases in liver blood flow resulting from the administration of β-adrenoceptor antagonists can reduce the metabolism of drugs such as verapamil and lidocaine. These drugs are rapidly removed from the circulation by the liver (high-extraction drugs) and their metabolism is therefore altered by changes in liver blood flow.

Inhibition of intestinal P-glycoprotein

P-glycoprotein is an important modulator of intestinal drug transport and functions to expel drugs from the intestinal mucosa into the lumen. Certain components of grapefruit juice inhibit the protein, which can result in higher concentrations of drugs that are excreted via this pathway – nifedipine, verapamil, ciclosporin, simvastatin.

Toxic metabolism

Some drugs are converted to toxic metabolites that can cause severe organ damage. In large doses a cytochrome P450-dependent system converts paracetamol to a reactive intermediate (N-acetyl-*p*-benzoquinoneimine) (see page 295 for more details).

Pharmacokinetics

Pharmacokinetics is the mathematical description of absorption, distribution and elimination of drugs in the body. The information gained from pharmacokinetic studies can be used to design dosage regimens and alter the formulation of a drug, eg in the production of long-acting preparations. Pharmacokinetics can also be used to aid the safe and effective management of patients who are receiving drugs with a narrow therapeutic index – aminoglycoside antibiotics, lithium, ciclosporin and phenytoin. The most important concepts in pharmacokinetics are:

- Effective drug concentration
- Clearance
- Apparent volume of distribution
- Elimination half-life
- Bioavailability
- Loading dose
- Maintenance dose

Effective drug concentration

The effective drug concentration is the concentration of a drug at its site of action that will produce the desired pharmacological effect. The subject of pharmacokinetics assumes that the concentration in the plasma mirrors the concentration at the receptor, and that measurement of the plasma concentration provides a more accurate assessment than the dose administered. For a small number of drugs this is the case, but for many compounds there is no clear relationship between plasma concentrations and effect.

Clearance

Clearance relates the rate of elimination to the plasma concentration:

$$\text{Clearance (Cl) (volume/time)} = \frac{\text{Rate of elimination (mass/time)}}{\text{Plasma drug concentration (mass/volume)}}$$

It can also be defined as the volume of plasma from which a drug is totally removed per unit time. The greater the concentration of the drug in the plasma, the greater the elimination of that drug (Figure 1.4). In first-order kinetics, the clearance is constant regardless of the plasma concentration and can vary from a small fraction of the total blood flow to a maximum of the total blood flow to the organ eliminating the drug.

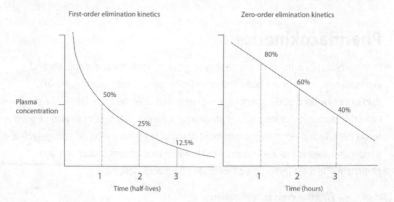

Figure 1.4 A comparison of first- and zero-order elimination kinetics. For first-order kinetics the rate of elimination is proportional to the concentration in the plasma and depends on the half-life. For zero-order kinetics the elimination is at a constant rate, independent of the plasma concentration, and its half-life cannot be defined.

Total body clearance is the sum of the clearances from the various organs involved in drug metabolism and elimination:

$$Cl_{total} = Cl_{renal} + Cl_{hepatic} + Cl_{extrarenal} + Cl_{extrahepatic}.$$

Note that students often find the concept of clearance difficult. It is not the same as elimination and its units are volume per unit time. Clearance is like a filter in an aquarium. The filter cleans a fixed amount of water in the aquarium in a given amount of time. The clean water returns to the aquarium, diluting the remaining water.

Apparent volume of distribution

The apparent volume of distribution relates the amount of drug in the body to its plasma concentration. It assumes that the drug is evenly distributed and that elimination has not taken place:

$$\text{Volume of distribution } (V_D) = \frac{\text{Amount of drug in the body}}{\text{Plasma concentration at time zero}}$$

An alternative definition would be the volume of plasma into which a drug appears to be diluted at a concentration equal to that in the plasma.

The greater the amount of drug outside the vascular compartment, the larger the apparent volume of distribution. A drug could be very lipid soluble and stored in fat or bound to plasma or tissue proteins. As a result, the apparent volume of distribution is usually larger than the plasma volume and often greater than total body fluid (Figure 1.5). It has no direct physical equivalent but can be used to define the loading dose of a drug and can be altered by liver disease (reduced protein synthesis), renal disease (protein loss) and the presence of other drugs (protein and tissue displacement). Drugs with large volumes of distribution are eliminated more slowly from the body than drugs with small volumes of distribution.

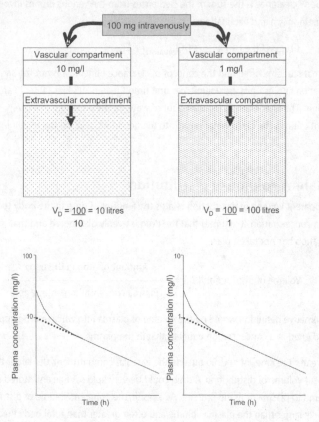

Figure 1.5 Drugs with small and large volumes of distribution. Plasma concentrations are lower when the volume of distribution is large.

Elimination half-life

The elimination half-life depends on the clearance and the apparent volume of distribution. A large volume of distribution and a low clearance result in a long elimination half-life whereas a small volume of distribution and a high clearance result in a short half-life.

$$\text{Elimination half-life} = 0.693 \times V_D/Cl$$

Disease, age and other factors usually alter the clearance more than the volume of distribution. The half-life determines the rate at which plasma drug concentrations increase and fall during maintenance dosing.

After 3.3 half-lives, 90% of steady state is achieved and, after 5 half-lives, 97% of steady state is achieved. By the same reasoning, only 3% of a drug will be present in the plasma 5 half-lives after a drug is discontinued.

Zero-order kinetics

When drugs saturate their routes of elimination (usually metabolism), removal from the body occurs at a fixed rate (see Figure 1.4). This is called 'zero-order kinetics' and applies to a large number of drugs taken in overdose. Three common examples of drugs that saturate liver metabolism within the therapeutic range are aspirin, phenytoin and alcohol. Alternative names for zero-order kinetics are non-linear or dose-dependent elimination.

Bioavailability

The bioavailability is the fraction of an administered drug dose that reaches the systemic circulation. After intravenous administration the bioavailability is defined as 100%. After administration by other routes bioavailability is usually reduced because of incomplete absorption and, in the case of the gut, first-pass metabolism and intestinal expulsion using a P-glycoprotein transporter. Even for drugs of equivalent bioavailability, entry into the systemic circulation varies with time depending on drug formulation, enterohepatic recirculation, alteration in gastric emptying and intestinal motility. To allow for this, the concentration appearing in the plasma is integrated over time using the area under the plasma concentration time curve. Oral bioavailability is then defined as:

$$\text{Bioavailability} = \frac{\text{Area under the curve (oral)}}{\text{Area under the curve (i.v.)}}$$

Loading dose

If the volume of distribution of a drug is large and its therapeutic concentration must be achieved rapidly, a loading dose may be required at the beginning of treatment. Examples include digoxin and amiodarone.

$$\text{Loading dose} = \frac{\text{Volume of distribution} \times \text{Desired plasma concentration}}{\text{Bioavailability}}$$

Maintenance dose

At steady state the amount of drug entering the body is equal to the amount leaving it. The maintenance dose is therefore a function of clearance and not of the volume of distribution.

$$\text{Dosing rate} = \frac{\text{Clearance} \times \text{Desired plasma concentration}}{\text{Bioavailability}}$$

A simple rule of thumb, however, which would result in trough concentrations that are 50% of peak concentrations, would be half the loading dose every half-life (Figure 1.6).

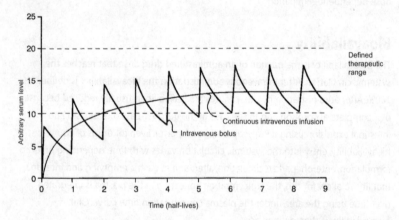

Figure 1.6 Relationship between maximum and minimum plasma concentrations (peak and trough) before and at steady state after intravenous boluses given each half-life. The effect of giving a continuous infusion to achieve the same steady-state plasma concentration is illustrated.

Pharmacodynamics

Pharmacodynamics deals with the effects of drugs in all biological systems. This can range from laboratory experiments involving isolated receptors to patients with specific diseases. Students should be aware of a number of definitions and concepts relating to how drugs produce their pharmacological effect.

Receptors

A receptor can be defined as a specific component of a biological system to which a drug binds to produce a functional change within that system. Receptors are selective in their ligand-binding characteristics and respond in a consistent manner to alterations imposed by a drug. The majority of receptors are proteins and a few are other macromolecules such as DNA. The receptor site is the specific binding region of the macromolecule and has a selective affinity for the drug molecule. This interaction is fundamental to the action of a drug.

Effectors

Effectors are molecules that translate the drug–receptor interaction into an alteration in cellular activity. The best known examples are enzymes such as adenylyl cyclase. Some receptors also function as effectors and incorporate drug-receptor binding with the effector mechanism. Examples include the tyrosine kinase effector of the insulin receptor and the Na^+/K^+ channel of the acetylcholine receptor.

Agonists

An agonist is a drug that binds to a receptor and produces activation of that receptor. A partial agonist is one that binds to the receptor but produces a smaller effect than a full agonist at maximum dosage.

Antagonists

An antagonist is a drug that binds to its receptor but does not result in activation. A competitive antagonist is a pharmacological antagonist that can be overcome by increasing the amount of the agonist. An irreversible or non-competitive antagonist is one that cannot be overcome by increasing the dose of an agonist. A physiological antagonist is a drug that reduces the effects of another by binding to a different receptor and producing the opposite effects. A chemical antagonist, on the other hand, is one that counters the effects of another agonist by binding to the drug and preventing its action.

Dose–response relationships

If the response of a receptor effector system is plotted against the drug concentration or dose, a graded dose–response curve is obtained. A standard sigmoid curve is obtained if the dose (or concentration) is plotted on a log scale.

Efficacy or, more correctly, maximal efficacy (E_{max}) can then be defined (Figure 1.7). Partial agonists have lower maximal efficacy than full agonists. Potency, on the other hand, denotes the amount of drug needed to produce a given effect. It is usually chosen as 50% of the maximal effect (EC_{50}) and is on the straight part of the log dose–response relationship (Figure 1.7). Potency is determined mainly by the affinity of the receptor for the drug and is a measure of the amount of the drug required to produce a pharmacological effect, eg as a diuretic, 1 mg bumetanide and 40 mg furosemide are equivalent in clinical practice and so bumetanide has greater potency; 1 mg bumetanide and 40 mg furosemide have equivalent efficacy, however.

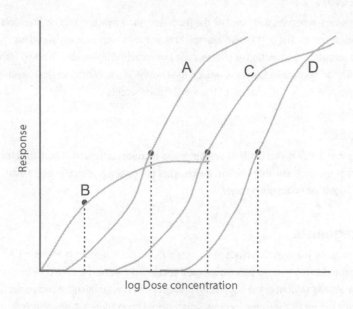

Figure 1.7 Dose–response relationships. Potency: drugs A and B are more potent than C and D because smaller doses are required to produce 50% of maximum effect (ED_{50}). Efficacy: drugs A, C and D have equal maximum efficacy, which is greater than that of B. Curve D represents a steep dose–response relationship compared with A, B and C. The responses at the top of this curve may be excessive and cause clinical problems, eg coma resulting from a sedative drug. (Alternatively the EC_{50} can be used, ie the plasma concentration required to produce 50% of maximum effect.) (Reproduced from Kenakin TP, Bond RA, Bonner TI. Definition of pharmacological receptors. *Pharmacological Reviews* 1992; **44**: 351-62, with permission of the American Society for Pharmacology and Experimental Therapeutics.)

Therapeutic index

When the minimum doses required to produce therapeutic and toxic responses are determined in population studies, the median effective dose (ED_{50}) and median lethal dose (LD_{50}) can be defined (Figure 1.8).

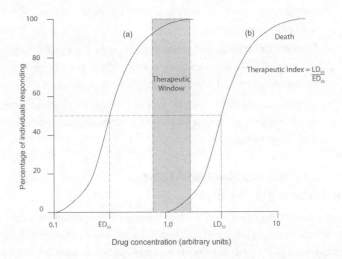

Figure 1.8 Concentration–response curves in the therapeutic (a) and toxic (b) ranges. The ED_{50} is the dose that will achieve a 50% response and the LD_{50} is the dose that will kill 50% of the animals receiving that dose.

The therapeutic index is the ratio of the LD_{50} to the ED_{50}. This represents an estimate of drug safety. A drug such as benzylpenicillin, which has a very large toxic dose and a low effective dose, is said to have a large or wide therapeutic index. Digoxin, on the other hand, has a low toxic dose that is close to its therapeutic dose and has a narrow therapeutic index. Careful therapeutic monitoring is therefore much more important for drugs that have a low or narrow therapeutic index.

Receptor classification

Receptors have been classed in a number of ways:

- According to the principal endogenous agonist that activates them – eg adrenoceptors (adrenaline), cholinoreceptors (acetylcholine).

- According to the first agonist found to activate them, often before an endogenous agonist has been discovered – eg opioid receptors, benzodiazepine receptors.

- Subclassification based on the rank order of potency of a series of agonists and the ability of antagonists to bind more avidly to one subtype of a receptor – histamine H_1 and H_2 receptors, β_1 and β_2 receptors.

- Definition according to molecular structure and function – ligand-gated ion channels, G-protein-coupled receptors, enzyme-linked receptors and DNA-linked receptors.

Regulation of receptors and their transduction mechanisms

For most drug–receptor interactions, the drug is present in the extracellular space and the effector system is present within the cell where it modifies the intracellular processes. Almost all processes therefore require transmembrane signalling and five potential mechanisms have been identified (Figure 1.9):

1. *Receptors present within the cell:* some lipid-soluble or diffusible agents may cross the membrane and combine with the intracellular receptor, eg steroid hormones.

2. *Receptors present on membrane-spanning enzymes:* molecules combine with a receptor on the extracellular portion of enzymes and modify its intracellular activity, eg insulin.

3. *Receptors present on membrane-spanning molecules:* after activation of the extracellular component of the receptor molecule, tyrosine kinase molecules are activated and produce 'STAT' molecules, which then travel to the nucleus where they regulate transcription.

4. *Receptors present on membrane ion channels:* drugs can act on receptors that regulate membrane ion channels and directly induce the opening of the channels, eg acetylcholine receptors, or modify the ion channel's response to other molecules, eg benzodiazepines at the γ-aminobutyric acid (GABA) channel (see page 131). This results in a change in the transmembrane electrical potential.

5. *Receptors linked to effectors via G-proteins:* a large number of drugs bind to receptors that are linked by coupling proteins to intracellular or membrane effectors. Adrenoceptor agonists and antagonists modulate adenylyl cyclase by a multistep process that involves interaction with the receptor and activation of G-proteins that either stimulate or inhibit the enzyme.

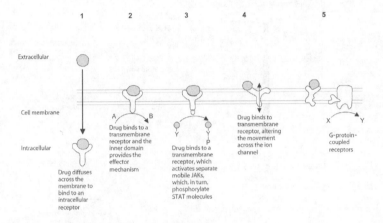

Figure 1.9 Major receptor signalling mechanisms.

Structure and function of the autonomic nervous system

Some background knowledge of the structure and function of the autonomic nervous system (ANS) is essential because a large number of cardiovascular, central nervous system (CNS) and respiratory drugs interact with this system.

Anatomy

The peripheral nervous system is divided into two branches: the somatic and autonomic nervous systems. The somatic system deals with voluntary muscle control whereas the ANS is responsible for maintaining the internal environment of the body and is largely involuntary.

Within the ANS, two neurones are required to reach the target organ: a preganglionic neurone and a postganglionic neurone (Figure 1.10). The preganglionic neurone originates within the CNS and forms a synapse with the postganglionic neurone, the cell body of which is present in the autonomic ganglion. All preganglionic neurones release the neurotransmitter acetylcholine, which binds to the nicotinic receptors in the postganglionic cell.

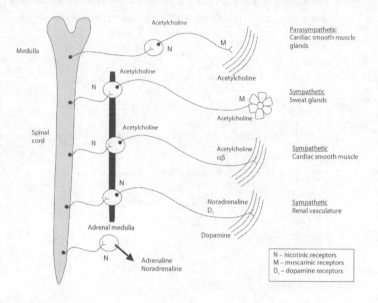

Figure 1.10 Examples of the different types of autonomic neurones, their related neurotransmitters and effector systems.

The ANS is divided into the sympathetic and parasympathetic systems. The sympathetic nerves arise from the thoroacolumbar plexus and have short preganglionic and long postganglionic fibres. This division of the ANS is catabolic (energy consuming) and is involved in the 'fight or flight response'. The parasympathetic nervous system is anabolic (energy conserving) and the preganglionic neurones are found in the brainstem (cranial nerves III, VII, IX, XII) and sacral outflow from the spinal cord (S2–4). The ganglia of the parasympathetic system are situated near the target organs so that the preganglionic neurones are long and the postganglionic neurones short. Within the parasympathetic system, one presynaptic axon usually forms a synapse with one or two postganglionic cells. The parasympathetic system therefore tends to be more localised in its mode of action. All parasympathetic neurones release acetylcholine and stimulate the muscarinic receptors at the target organ. Most sympathetic postganglionic fibres release noradrenaline (norepinephrine), which stimulates a variety of different receptors at the target organ. Sweat glands are supplied by sympathetic cholinergic nerves. The adrenal medulla is also part of the sympathetic nervous system and release of adrenaline and noradrenaline into the systemic circulation plays an important role in the 'fight or flight' response.

Neurotransmitter aspects of the ANS

Most drugs that affect the ANS act at receptors, but some alter the synthesis, storage, release and degradation of autonomic neurotransmitters.

Cholinergic transmission

Acetylcholine is the neurotransmitter at all autonomic ganglia, all postganglionic parasympathetic synapses and some postganglionic sympathetic synapses (Figure 1.11).

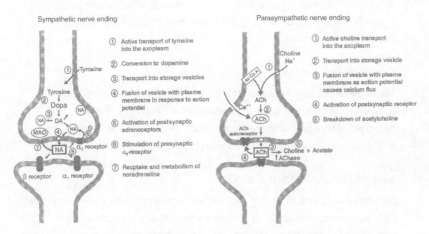

Figure 1.11 Comparison of the stages involved in neurotransmitter synthesis and metabolism at the sympathetic and parasympathetic nerve endings.

Synthesis and storage

Acetylcholine is synthesised from acetyl-CoA and choline by the enzyme choline acetyltransferase. Hemicholinium inhibits the synthesis of acetylcholine and vesamicol prevents its storage.

Release of acetylcholine

Botulinum toxin inhibits the release of acetylcholine from the vesicles at the nerve ending. This effect is most commonly seen at the neuromuscular synapse, resulting in paralysis of striated muscle.

Termination of action of acetylcholine

Acetylcholinesterase is responsible for the termination of action of acetylcholine by converting it to choline and acetate. Inhibition of this enzyme is the mode of action of anticholinesterase inhibitors, eg neostigmine, which are used to treat myasthenia gravis. The acute toxic effects of organophosphate insecticides are also caused by inhibition of acetylcholinesterase.

Adrenergic transmission

Noradrenaline is the neurotransmitter at postganglionic neurone–effector cell synapses in most tissues. Acetylcholine is the neurotransmitter for sympathetic neurones to sweat glands and probably to vasodilator fibres in skeletal muscle (Figure 1.11). Dopamine is an important vasodilator transmitter in renal blood vessels.

Synthesis and storage

The synthesis of noradrenaline involves the hydroxylation of tyrosine to dopa (dihydroxyphenylalanine), which is decarboxylated to dopamine and then hydroxylated to noradrenaline within the vesicle (Figure 1.11). Reserpine, a centrally acting antihypertensive agent, inhibits transport into the vesicle.

Release and termination of action

Noradrenaline and dopamine are released from their nerve endings in stored vesicles in a similar manner to acetylcholine. However, in contrast, metabolism is not responsible for their inactivation. Concentrations in the synaptic cleft are reduced by diffusion and reuptake. Outside the cleft, metabolism takes place by monoamine oxidase (MAO) and catechol-O-methyltransferase (COMT). Guanethidine and related compounds lower blood pressure by inhibiting the release of noradrenaline into the synaptic cleft, whereas cocaine and tricyclic antidepressants block the reuptake of noradrenaline at the nerve endings. Phenelzine, which is used in the treatment of major depression, and selegiline, which is used to treat Parkinson's disease, inhibit the enzyme MAO.

Adrenoceptors

Receptors for noradrenaline are divided into α and β receptors. These are further subdivided into α_1 and α_2 and β_1, β_2 and β_3. The most important site for β_1 is the heart, for β_2 the bronchial smooth muscle and skeletal muscle blood vessels, and for β_3 adipose tissue. The α-receptors are present in smooth muscle. Their location and major functions are listed in Table 1.4. Dopamine receptors are a subclass of adrenoceptors, and have important roles in the regulation of vascular function in the kidney, brain and gut. Four subtypes have been identified: D_1, D_2, D_3 and D_4. D_1 receptors are the most important peripheral effector-cell receptors; D_2 receptors are found on presynaptic nerve terminals; and D_3 and D_4 receptors have important effects on the cerebral circulation.

Receptor	Location	Major functions
$\alpha 1$	Smooth muscle Glands	Increases calcium with cells causing contraction and secretion
$\alpha 2$	Nerve endings Smooth muscle	Inhibits noradrenaline release. Causes contraction
$\beta 1$	Cardiac muscle Kidney	Increases heart rate, and force of contraction. Increases renin release
$\beta 2$	Smooth muscle Cardiac muscle	Relaxes smooth muscle. Increases gluconeogenesis. Increases heart rate and force of contraction
$\beta 3$	Adipose tissue	Increases lipolysis

Table 1.4 Characteristics of the main adrenoceptors in the ANS

Cholinoreceptors (Table 1.5)

There are two major classes of receptors for acetylcholine: muscarinic and nicotinic. Muscarinic receptors are located principally on autonomic effector cells in the heart, vascular endothelium, smooth muscle, presynaptic nerve terminals and exocrine glands. Evidence has been found for five subtypes and three are important for peripheral autonomic transmission – M_1, M_2 and M_3.

Receptor	Location	Major functions
M_1	Nerve endings	↑ IP_3
M_2	Heart, some nerve endings	↓ cAMP
M_3	Effector cells, glands, smooth muscle endothelium	↑ IP_3

cAMP, cyclic adenosine 3':5'-monophosphate; IP_3, 1,4,5-inositol triphosphate.

Table 1.5 Characteristics of the main cholinoreceptors in the ANS

The two main types of nicotinic receptor are located in the autonomic ganglia and skeletal muscle end-plates. The nicotinic receptors are the primary receptors for transmission at these sites.

Autonomic innervation: maintaining a balance

General rules (Table 1.6)

Organ	Responses			
	Sympathetic		Parasympathetic	
	Action	Receptor	Action	Receptor
Eye (iris)				
Radial muscle	Contracts	α_1	Contracts	M_3
Circular muscle	—	—	Contracts	M_3
Ciliary muscle	[Relaxes]	β		
Heart				
Sinoatrial node	Accelerates	$\beta_1 \beta_2$	Slows	M_2
Contractility	Increases	$\beta_1 \beta_2$	Decreases	M_2
Blood vessels				
Skin/splanchnic	Contracts	α		
Skeletal muscle	Relaxes	β_2		
Endothelium			Releases nitric oxide	M_3
Lungs				
Bronchial smooth muscle	Relaxes	β_2	Contracts	M_3
Gut				
Wall	Relaxes	$\alpha_2 \beta_2$	Contracts	M_3
Sphincter	Contracts	α_1	Relaxes	M_3
Secretion			Increases	$M_1 M_3$

Table 1.6 Principal actions of the sympathetic and parasympathetic nervous systems

- For most organs innervated by the sympathetic and parasympathetic systems, the two systems have opposing actions.

- Structures receiving this dual nerve supply include the heart, eye and smooth muscle of the gastrointestinal, bronchial and genitourinary tracts.

- In the vegetative or resting state, the predominant influence is from the parasympathetic system.

- Most vascular smooth muscle is innervated exclusively by the sympathetic nervous system. Maintenance of blood pressure and peripheral resistance therefore depends on the activity of the sympathetic nervous system, and many effective antihypertensive agents prevent vasoconstriction.

- Contraction of radial smooth muscle of the iris causes dilatation and mydriasis, a function of the sympathetic nervous system. Stimulation of the parasympathetic system causes contraction of circular smooth muscle and miosis.

- Activation of α-receptors causes smooth muscle contraction and vasoconstriction.

- The heart is the main site for β_1 receptors and β_2 receptors occur in the airways.

2

Principles of therapeutics

2 Principles of therapeutics

Drug therapeutics is much more than the matching of a drug to a disease. It requires knowledge, judgement, skill and experience, together with a strong sense of responsibility. Several factors come into play when a patient receives a medication that are unrelated to the action of a drug or the nature of the disease. Examples include: the patient's and doctor's attitude and demeanour at the time of prescribing; the personality and beliefs of both parties; the expectations of the patient; and his or her previous experience of the medical profession.

Is drug therapy the preferred option?

Before embarking on drug therapy a number of points should be borne in mind. If a drug is chosen, does it represent the most appropriate treatment option and is it likely to achieve the best therapeutic result? What is the best way to administer the drug, can the effects be measured, does the drug have important adverse effects and when should it be discontinued?

Balancing benefits and risk

Poisons in small doses are the best medicines; and useful medicines in too large doses are poisonous.

Withering (1785) An Account of the Foxglove and its medical uses.

Individualisation of Drug Therapy

After choosing the most suitable drug based on the best available information, the therapist has to determine the most appropriate dosage regimen. Variation between and within patients must be taken into account. For some drugs this variation can be very large. In general, drugs which undergo extensive metabolism show greater variation than those which are excreted unchanged in the urine. Drugs with low oral bioavailability also demonstrate greater variability than those which are well absorbed and/or not subject to first pass metabolism. Impaired liver and renal function as a result of disease or age will delay the excretion of drugs which are eliminated by these routes. Reduced doses will be required in these patients. Disease can also alter the responsiveness to certain drugs. For example, the inotropic effect of digoxin increases with the severity of heart failure and vasodilator drugs increase cardiac output in this condition while having the opposite effect in normal subjects. In diabetes the action of sulphonylureas, which stimulate the beta receptors in the pancreas, depends on the number of receptors and in type 11 diabetes the effect on blood glucose concentrations decreases with time as the number of receptors decline.

Adjustment of dosage should be made, if possible, on the clinical response to treatment. However, for some drugs in certain clinical settings effects are not easily monitored. Control of the ventricular rate in atrial fibrillation can be assessed but if digoxin is used in patients with heart failure and sinus rhythm plasma drug monitoring is also difficult for drugs which are used in prophylaxis ego anticonvulsant therapy. Estimation of steady state plasma concentrations of anticonvulsants can be useful to avoid toxicity and check for non-compliance with drug treatment.

Benefits

The benefits of drug therapy can be summarised under three headings: cure, prevention and symptomatic treatment.

Cure

This is sometimes achieved, eg when treating bacterial or parasitic disease, the disease is often eliminated after drug withdrawal. Anaesthetic agents, and drugs used to induce and maintain labour also result in beneficial effects after drug withdrawal and can be considered 'curative'.

Prevention

This is usually divided into primary and secondary:

Primary prevention is when a treatment aims to prevent a healthy person getting a disease. Examples include malaria prophylaxis, immunisations, and the use of statins to prevent cardiovascular disease.

In *secondary prevention*, the patient has a disease and treatment is targeted to reduce risk factors and retard progression of the disease. Important examples include aspirin, antihypertensives and lipid-lowering therapy to prevent atherosclerosis and its clinical manifestations, after a patient has had a myocardial infarction or stroke.

Symptomatic treatment

This is the use of drugs to control symptoms while awaiting recovery from the causative disease or to suppress symptoms of a chronic disease. Examples include the treatment of asthma, epilepsy, chronic pain, and palliative care.

Risks

Drugs can cause harm for a variety of reasons:

- *Lack of selectivity:* action at receptor sites other than the target results in unwanted action, eg bronchospasm resulting from blockade of β_2-adrenoceptors in the lung by β-adrenoceptor antagonists.
- *Different effects in different organs:* a drug with a beneficial effect at one site can cause adverse effects at another, eg inhibition of cyclo-oxygenase to reduce prostaglandin formation in an inflamed joint can cause gastrointestinal bleeding and renal impairment by a similar mechanism in different organs.
- *Insufficient knowledge of drug action:* when a drug is introduced, adverse effects may develop by mechanisms that were not predicted by the known action of the drug, eg the cough induced by angiotensin-converting enzyme (ACE) inhibitors and the increased incidence of sudden death caused by anti-arrhythmic and inotropic drugs.
- *Prolonged modification of cellular mechanisms:* this can result in permanent structural and functional change, eg carcinogenicity.
- *Genetic predisposition:* patients may be at increased risk of adverse effects because of reduced metabolism. Slow acetylators and slow oxidisers have a genetic abnormality that increases their risk of adverse events when certain drugs are prescribed. Patients with glucose-6-phosphate dehydrogenase (G6PD) deficiency can develop haemolysis when a variety of drugs are given.
- *Insufficient dose adjustment for renal or hepatic impairment.*
- *Ignorance and casual prescribing.*

The risk of adverse effects can be reduced by modification of the drug therapy, molecular manipulation, specific drug targeting, and careful and responsible prescribing. Despite these measures, drugs will continue to do harm. It has been suggested that when risks fall below 1 in 100 000, the treatment (or procedure) can be considered as 'safe'. When individuals develop rare adverse effects, however, it is often difficult for them to accept this concept, and they are likely to blame the doctor or manufacturer, when in actual fact there has been no fault or negligence.

Grades of risk

These can be divided into unacceptable, acceptable and negligible. In all these cases, however, the risks cannot be viewed in isolation and must be related to potential benefit. Unfortunately there are often insufficient data available to ensure a rational decision about drug therapy in every case. These decisions have to be made during the consultation process. In some chronic diseases, such as hypertension, the patient may be little inconvenienced by the disease and may prefer not to take drugs, although the later manifestations of the condition may be catastrophic. In these circumstances it can often be difficult to persuade patients to take drug therapy.

Medication errors

It is estimated that between 44 000 and 98 000 Americans die each year from medical errors and more than a million experience significant adverse events. About half of these are related to drug therapy, and of the serious adverse events, about 50% are preventable. There are a number of areas that could be addressed to improve the present situation:

- Improved knowledge and prescribing ability of doctors
- More balanced promotion of new drugs by the pharmaceutical industry and fewer financial incentives for the prescriber
- Informed discussion of drug prescribing by the media, medical profession, pharmaceutical industry, patients and politicians
- Introduction of 'no fault' compensation schemes for serious drug injury.

'No fault' compensation

There is a growing view that compensation is required for serious personal injury, which should be automatic and not dependent on fault or proof of fault. This is defined as 'no fault' compensation. Drugs represent a class of product for which there has been the greatest pressure to introduce this form of compensation. It would reduce the number of cases of litigation against doctors in which negligence has to be proved, and patients would be automatically compensated for their injuries.

Economic factors

Reducing the amount of money spent on medications attracts increasing attention, particularly from politicians and civil servants. It largely involves two contentious activities promoted by health authorities and opposed by the pharmaceutical industry.

Generic substitution

Generic formulations are substituted for proprietary ('trade-name') formulations. Generic formulations cost less and there is little evidence that they are inferior to the proprietary preparations. Pharmaceutical companies complain that they have spent considerable sums of money developing and researching their products, only to be undercut by other companies (which have not incurred these costs) producing the generic preparation. Some manufacturers produce 'slow-release' preparations or make minor modifications to the original compound to extend the 'marketable' life of their product.

Therapeutic substitution

Drugs of different chemical structures are substituted for the prescribed drug. The drug is in the same chemical class, eg enalapril substituted for perindopril, and can be expected to produce the same pharmacological effect. Therapeutic substitution is a very controversial area, especially if it is instigated without the knowledge of the prescriber, and legal issues may ensue if an adverse outcome or event results.

It is important that the incentives and sanctions introduced in these schemes address quality issues as well as quantity. There is a real danger that these incentive schemes could result in under-prescribing, particularly of drugs used in primary and secondary prevention.

Pharmacoeconomics

There are four economic concepts that are important to every doctor who prescribes medications:

1. Opportunity cost

This depends on the fact that spending on health will always be finite. If more money is spent on drug prescribing, money will not be available for other purposes, eg money saved by generic prescribing could be used for institutionalised mentally handicapped patients.

2. Cost-effectiveness analysis

This is a measure of how the cost of a drug and its adverse effects relates to the financial benefits of using the drug, and includes items such as materials, nursing and doctor time, diagnostic tests and length of stay in hospital.

3. Cost–benefit analysis

This assessment puts monetary value on quality and duration of life as well as on the items included in the cost-effectiveness analysis. It is currently used to influence Government policy on health care and is included in the deliberations of the National Institute for Health and Clinical Excellence (NICE) and the Scottish Medicines Consortium (SMC) for their adjudications on new therapeutic interventions.

4. Cost–utility analysis

This is a general measure of improved quality of life and seeks to obtain a measure that can be applied to all diseases and age groups. The measurement most frequently used is the QALY (quality-adjusted life-year). It is assessed using questionnaires to measure what the individual perceives as personal health and has four principal dimensions:

- Physical mobility
- Freedom from pain and distress
- Capacity for self-care and ability to engage in normal work
- Social interactions.

Drug compliance

Patient compliance is the extent to which the behaviour of the patient coincides with medical advice and instruction. It is usually measured as the ratio of the amount of drug taken by the patient (measured by tablet counts, plasma or urine samples, or electronic monitoring) to the amount that was prescribed. It may be complete, partial, erratic or absent. Between 5% and 20% of all prescriptions are not presented to the pharmacist for dispensing. Some 25–50% of patients fail to follow instructions and take less or more than the prescribed dose. The two main situations where non-compliance occurs are when the patient does not understand the instructions or does understand but fails or refuses to carry them out. Factors that have been shown to relate to non-compliance include the complexity of the drug regimen, forgetfulness, lack of information, poor doctor–patient relationship, impaired motivation and wilful non-compliance. Poor drug compliance is the most important reason why patients fail to respond to drug therapy.

An alternative view of patient–doctor behaviour is encapsulated in the term 'concordance'. The concept is particularly important in explaining intelligent or wilful non-compliance, and the factors relating to impaired motivation and understanding. Concordance is a method of assessing whether the patient's health beliefs and the doctor's decisions to treat are compatible. If the patient's views are at variance with that of the prescriber's, the patient is likely to be non-compliant. The most successful doctor–patient relationships will be those in which the views of both parties on the disease and its treatment are as similar as possible, ie concordant.

Placebo medicines

Placebo medications are used in medicine for two purposes: as a control in clinical trials and, occasionally, to please the patient by psychological rather than pharmacological means. Most prefer the term 'dummy' rather than 'placebo' in clinical trials because there is no intent to 'please' the patient. All treatments have a psychological component to enhance or reduce the therapeutic effect. The deliberate use of drugs as placebos is a confession of failure by the doctor, although the prescribing of vitamins and other supplements as tonics is relatively harmless. There are two main groups of patients who cause problems for drug prescribers. Firstly, there are suggestible patients who respond favourably to any treatment. Such prescribing can have clear benefit to the patient, but has misled doctors into making false therapeutic claims. The other patients who can also cause problems for long-term management are the 'negative' placebo reactors, who develop adverse effects when given a placebo and complain of a number of non-specific adverse effects when given any medication.

Complementary or alternative medicine

The realisation by the population that modern medicine cannot guarantee happiness or wholly eliminate disease, and can cause serious adverse effects, has resulted in a revival of alternative therapies that promise benefit without adverse effects.

Features of complementary medicine are those that bedevilled conventional medicine before the development of rational and scientific thinking. Such ideas include naïve acceptance of untested hypotheses, uncritical acceptance of causation, reliance on anecdote, and the assumption that if the patient recovers it is as a result of the treatment given. An important spiritual ritualistic or magical dimension is a feature of most complementary therapies and may serve to enhance the placebo effect in susceptible individuals. Commonly held views by alternative practitioners on modern medicine are that modern drugs are toxic but natural products are not, that scientific medicine rests on acceptance of rigid dogmas and that only treatments for which the mechanisms of action are known can be used to treat patients. Views on alternative medicine include: traditional medicines have a special (or spiritual) dimension; it is not necessary to collect information on therapeutic outcomes – failure and successes; and the belief that, if a patient gets better in accordance with certain beliefs, it provides evidence for the truth of those beliefs (the *post hoc ergo propter hoc* fallacy).

Attempts to subject alternative treatment to scientific assessment have been made but most studies lack statistical power and/or have significant design flaws. Meta-analyses of complementary therapies mainly conclude that the beneficial effects are comparable to those of placebo. There remain, however, a group of practitioners who reject the scientific assessment of their treatments and state that their beliefs are not refutable. This has been the position of religion and magic throughout the centuries, where subordination of reason to faith has been considered a virtue.

Some of the criticisms made by alternative practitioners about modern medicine do, however, have an element of truth. There is a view that many practitioners of conventional medicine do not treat the patient's body, mind and spirit and, with the development of specialisation, some practitioners have become too narrow and preoccupied with the technological aspects of their work. Overall, complementary medicine does not compete with mainstream medicine in any significant way. Often it is used by those with chronic disease who have had little or no benefit from conventional treatment.

Discovery and development of medicines

Discovery

Almost all useful medications in the past were derived from plant and animal sources, aspirin form willow bark, opiates from the opium poppy and digitalis from the foxglove leaf and during the twentieth century the pharmacological revolution depended largely on the modification of existing, naturally occurring compounds. Sporadic attempts were made over the centuries to distinguish useful (rare) and useless (common) compounds, but none were successful as a result of the dominance of belief systems that purported to explain human biology and disease without experimentation and observation. At the end of the seventeenth century, observation and experimentation began to replace belief systems after the example of the physical sciences. *Materia medica*, the science of drug preparation and the medical use of drugs, began to develop as the forerunner of pharmacology. Advances in chemistry and physiology during the nineteenth and early twentieth centuries laid the foundation required for the understanding of drug action. From the middle of the last century, as new concepts and techniques were introduced, and information accumulated about the action of drugs, many novel useful compounds became available.

The evolution of molecular medicine in the past 20 years has resulted in a potentially fruitful area for drug discovery – pharmacogenomics. The chance of determining a truly novel medication is increased when the development programme is based on biological processes at a molecular level. Some of the claims for this branch of biology have been exaggerated, however, and it seems likely that the benefits will take longer to materialise than originally expected.

The application of scientific principles to the treatment of disease continues, but unfortunately the public continues to be exposed to large amounts of inaccurate, unscientific and incomplete information on the nature of drug therapy. This has resulted in the use of numerous expensive, ineffective and sometimes harmful remedies, and the growth of an enormous 'alternative' health-care industry.

Techniques of drug discovery

For details of this see Figure 2.1.

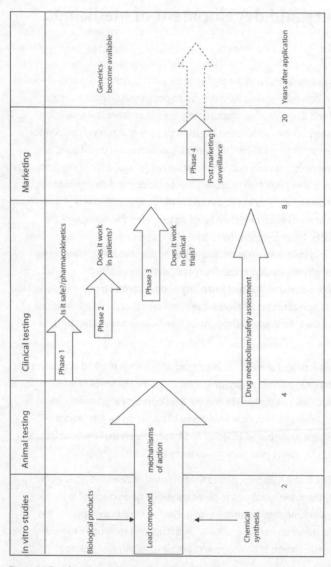

Figure 2.1 Development and testing process required to bring a new drug onto the market.

Sources of drug discovery

- Natural products: plants and animal sources.

- Traditional medicine: identifying the occasional wheat from the plentiful chaff.

- Modification of known drugs: these usually result in similar pharmacological properties but can cause a few surprises, eg sotalol, a β-adrenoceptor antagonist, has class I anti-arrhythmic activity, and practolol produced a unique adverse effect profile compared with other β antagonists.

- Random screening for natural products: the Amazon jungle, for example, is likely to be a fruitful source.

- New uses for old drugs: the use of aspirin for its antiplatelet rather than its anti-inflammatory activity is an obvious example.

- Molecular modelling: three-dimensional computer graphics allow the design of structures based on existing and new molecules to determine possible receptor interactions. The structure of the early angiotensin receptor antagonists relied on this technique.

- Combinational chemistry: this involves the synthesis of billions of compounds, usually based on amino acids, nucleotides or pharmacologically active compounds, to produce libraries that can then be subjected to robotic screening.

- Protein synthesis: as the targets of most drugs are proteins and many hormones are polypeptides, protein synthesis using bacteria or yeasts is, and will be, an important source of drugs.

- Gene therapy: the idea of delivering genes to deficient cells via viruses or other cell carriers has enormous potential in genetic conditions such as cystic fibrosis.

- Immunopharmacology.

Development

Drug development can be divided into five main stages:

1. Hypothesis, design and synthesis
2. Studies on tissues and whole animals (preclinical)
3. Studies in humans (clinical)
4. Licensing to market the compound
5. Post-marketing surveillance.

Pre-clinical studies in animals

Various pre-clinical studies are performed in animals to help reduce the risk of human toxicity, to explore the pharmacokinetics and pharmacodynamics, and to identify the likely starting dose. Various toxicological tests are performed, usually in rodents and dogs, which can last from 2 weeks to 12 months, as shown in Table 2.1.

Duration of the planned clinical trial		Minimum duration of repeat toxicity studies in animals required	
Type of trial	Who will be recruited?	Rodents	Non-rodents
Single dose	Volunteers	2 weeks	2 weeks
Up to 2 weeks	Volunteers Patients	2 weeks 1 month	2 weeks 1 month
Up to 1 month	Volunteers Patients	1 month 3 months	1 month 3 months
Up to 3 months	Volunteers Patients	3 months 6 months	3 months 3 months
> 3 months	Patients	6 months	(12) months*
Up to 6 months	Volunteers	6 months	6 months
> 6 months	Volunteers	6 months	(12) months*

*A 6-month study may be accepted on a case-by-case basis.

Table 2.1 The need for animal studies before clinical trials

Other tests include those for mutagenicity, eg the Ames test, potential chromosome damage and carcinogenicity testing which involves the whole animal for compounds in which the mutagenicity test is unsatisfactory. Reproduction studies include effects on fertility, reproductive function, fetal organogenesis and peri- and postnatal development, and are usually undertaken in rabbits. Later studies involve assessment of the growth, behaviour and intellectual function of the offspring. These are known as second-generation effects.

Clinical trials

Experiments in humans are divided into four phases: phases 1–3 are required for licensing the product, and phase 4 studies are conducted after a licence has been obtained.

Phase 1

A phase 1 trial consists of careful evaluation of the dose–response characteristics in a minimum of 20 healthy volunteers. The early pharmacokinetics and dynamics are assessed at the different dosages and minor toxic effects identified. For new anti-cancer drugs, these studies are performed in patients with cancer.

Phase 2

Phase 2 trials are undertaken in 50–300 patients with the target disease. A placebo or control drug is included in a single- or double-blind design. The principal aim is to determine whether the medication has the desired therapeutic effect at doses that are tolerated by sick patients.

Phase 3

A phase 3 trial seeks to confirm or refute the observations obtained in a phase 2 trial by assessing the drug in larger numbers of patients, often more than 1000. They are usually multicentre, employ several investigators and are double blind in design, with a placebo or matching drug. Their main role is to explore the actions of the drug, compare it with existing therapies and determine adverse effects.

Phase 4

This represents the post-marketing surveillance phase of drug evaluation in which rare adverse events can be identified and reported, aiming to prevent major harm to treated populations.

Pharmacoepidemiology

Pharmacoepidemiology is the study of the use and effects of drugs in large populations. Studies of this type are particularly useful for identifying adverse events that have been missed in phase 3 trials. These phase 4 trials rely on observational data and are used when large randomised trials are logistically and financially prohibitive. They can on occasions produce misleading results.

Observational cohort studies

In this type of study, patients receiving a drug are followed up to determine a therapeutic or adverse outcome. The trials need to be long-term, and comparisons are made with a suitable control group. A good example is prescription event monitoring, in which prescriptions are sent to a central pricing and payment authority. The prescriber is then sent a questionnaire and asked to report all clinical events that occur without any judgement on causality. Alternatively this can be reported electronically and can involve other health professionals – pharmacists, nurses or patients. By linking general practice and hospital records, unsuspected effects can be detected. This type of study is most suitable for new drugs that are widely prescribed.

Case–control studies

In this type of study the investigator assembles a group of patients who have a certain disease and compares them with a group of matched controls who do not have that disease. A factor may be identified in the 'disease' group, eg more patients with thromboembolic disease may take oral contraception compared with a 'healthy' control group. Case–control studies do not prove causation but show associations.

Pharmacovigilance

Pharmacovigilance is the process of identifying and responding to issues of drug safety by detecting potential adverse effects in treated populations. Although cohort and case–control studies are sometimes used, the process relies most heavily on voluntary reporting by doctors, pharmacists and nurses, who are supplied with cards to record adverse drug reactions. In the UK this is known as the 'Yellow Card Scheme' and the information is collated by the Medicines and Healthcare products Regulatory Agency (MHRA). Yellow cards are at the back of the *British National Formulary* and require doctors to report:

- All suspected reactions with new medicines – those identified in the BNF with an inverted black triangle ▼).
- Serious suspected reactions to established medicines – even if a well-recognised or causal link is uncertain.

Surveys suggest gross under-reporting of the system, especially if the adverse event takes time to develop. It cannot be used to determine the likely incidence of an adverse event but, overall, the system has been successful in detecting adverse events not reported in phase 3 trials.

Box 2.1 Definitions

Single-blind study: a clinical trial in which the investigator, but not the doctor or patient, is aware of which medication is being administered in a comparative study.

Double-blind study: a clinical trial in which neither investigators nor patients are aware of the medication that is being received. A code is held by a third party, and in large clinical outcome trials a safety committee is employed, which can stop the trial if impaired efficacy or increased toxicity is detected.

Positive control: a known standard therapy to be used with placebo to evaluate fully the safety and efficacy of the new medication in relation to what is currently available.

Orphan drug: a drug developed for a rare disease. Governments and charities may support the industry in developing these medications.

The null hypothesis: when comparing two treatments, the null hypothesis proposes that they are not different. If one treatment is better than the other, the null hypothesis is rejected.

Statistical significance: if there is a difference between two treatments that is likely to occur by chance with a frequency of < 1 in 20, the difference is said to be statistically significant ($p < 0.05$). A frequency of < 1 in 100 is usually reported as highly significant ($p < 0.01$).

Type I error: this occurs when a difference is found that is not a true difference, ie the null hypothesis has been rejected inappropriately.

Type II error: occurs when no difference has been found even though there is a true difference, ie the null hypothesis has been accepted inappropriately. It is likely to occur when the study lacks statistical power.

Box 2.1 Definitions *(continued)*

Statistical power: provides a measure of the probability of avoiding a type II error and detecting a real difference. Adequate power is often defined as giving an 80–90% chance of detecting a difference of 15% at a *p* value of < 0.05.

Meta-analysis: this type of analysis involves collecting a number of trials with the same objective and analysing the accumulated results.

Confidence intervals: the confidence interval expresses a range of values which includes the true value with 95% (or other chosen percentage, eg 99%) confidence. A wide confidence interval occurs when numbers are small and/or the individual differences are variable (see Figure 2.2).

Relative risk reduction: this represents a percentage reduction in the main outcome measure. If five people die in the treatment group and ten on placebo, this would represent a 50% reduction in mortality.

Absolute risk reduction: represents the number of lives saved or diseases prevented in the above example related to the population studied. The absolute risk reduction could be 5 per 1000, a less impressive statistic.

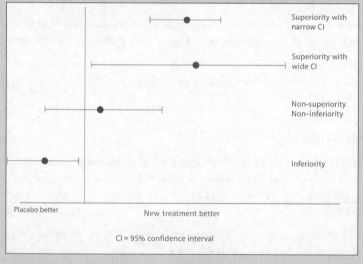

Figure 2.2 Illustration of confidence intervals in the comparison between a new treatment and placebo.

3
Cardiovascular system

Diuretics
Beta blockers
Calcium-channel blocking drugs
Alpha blockers
Angiotensin-converting enzyme inhibitors
Angiotensin II receptor antagonists
Organic nitrates
Inotropes
Thrombolytics
Anti-arrhythmic drugs
HMG-CoA reductase inhibitors
Fibric acid derivatives
Resins
Nicotinic acid
Management of acute MI
Management of acute left ventricular failure

3
Cardiovascular system

Diuretics

There are four main types of diuretics in common clinical use: thiazide, loop, potassium-sparing diuretics and aldosterone antagonists (Table 3.1). All three groups increase sodium and water excretion by the kidney, but act at different sites along the nephron as shown in Figure 3.1.

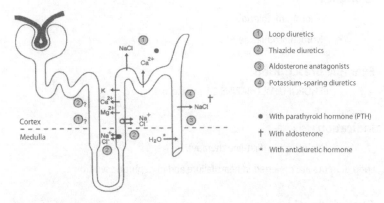

① Loop diuretics
② Thiazide diuretics
③ Aldosterone anatagonists
④ Potassium-sparing diuretics

● With parathyroid hormone (PTH)
† With aldosterone
* With antidiuretic hormone

Figure 3.1 Schematic diagram of a nephron showing the site of action of diuretics.

Thiazide	Loop	Potassium-sparing	Aldosterone anagonists
Bendroflumethiazide Hydrochlorothiazide	Furosemide Bumetamide	Amiloride Triamterene	Spironolactone

Table 3.1 Diuretics in clinical use

Thiazide diuretics

Mechanism of action

Thiazide diuretics act by inhibiting sodium and chloride co-transport across the luminal membrane in the cortical diluting segment of the distal convoluted tubule. Normally, 5–10% of the filtered sodium load is reabsorbed in this region. Thiazides are active by the oral route and most have a duration of action lasting 6–12 hours.

These drugs promote salt and water loss by the kidney. A reduction in intracellular sodium within the tubular cells increases Na^+/Ca^{2+} exchange and reduces loss of calcium from the tubule. The mechanism of the blood pressure-lowering effect is unknown but cannot be related to sodium loss, because low doses are as effective as high doses. A vasodilator effect has been proposed.

Examples

- Bendroflumethiazide
- Hydrochlorothiazide.

Example prescription

BENDROFLUMETHIAZIDE 2.5 mg p.o. o.d.

Indication

- Hypertension (first-line therapy).

Loop diuretics are preferred in heart failure and in nephrotic syndrome.

Contraindications

- Any of the 'fluid and electrolyte' side effects noted below
- Renal or hepatic impairment.

Common side effects (Table 3.2)

Fluid and electrolyte	Metabolic	Hypersensitivity
Hypovolaemia	Diabetes mellitus	Pancreatitis
Hypokalaemia	Hypercholesterolaemia	Nephritis
Hyponatraemia	Hyperuricaemia	Photosensitivity
Hypomagnesaemia		
Hypercalcaemia		

Table 3.2 Side effects of thiazide diuretics

Most adverse effects are dose-dependent. The risk of diabetes is greatest when thiazide diuretics are combined with β-blockers.

Significant interactions

For significant interactions of thiazide diuretics, see Table 3.3.

Drug	Interaction
Lithium	Reduced renal clearance of lithium and increased risk of lithium toxicity
Non-steroidal anti-inflammatory drugs	Reduced diuretic and antihypertensive effects
Angiotensin-converting enzyme (ACE) inhibitors	Prior use of diuretics predisposes to first-dose hypotension
Digoxin	Diuretic-induced hypokalaemia increases the risk of digoxin toxicity
Uricosuric agents and xanthine oxidase inhibitors (eg allopurinol)	Reduce the effectiveness of anti-gout medication
Aminoglycosides	Increase the risk of nephrotoxicity when administered together[*]

[*]Loop diuretics only.

Table 3.3 Interactions with loop and thiazide diuretics

Loop diuretics

Mechanism of action

Loop diuretics inhibit sodium and chloride reabsorption in the thick ascending loop of Henle. They are all actively secreted by the proximal tubule and achieve high concentrations at the luminal membrane of the loop of Henle. Acute vascular effects (venodilatation, increased renal blood flow and peripheral arteriolar constriction) have also been described, which occur before a diuresis is apparent.

Loop diuretics are most commonly used in the treatment of heart failure. They have a steep dose–response relationship and work in the presence of impaired renal function. Loop diuretics produce their benefit by reducing plasma volume and venous return to the heart. Intravenous furosemide or bumetanide produce these effects rapidly and, together with venodilatation, relieve breathlessness in acute pulmonary oedema.

Examples

- Furosemide
- Bumetanide.

Example prescription

FUROSEMIDE 40 mg i.v. o.d.

Indications

- Heart failure
- Ascites caused by chronic liver disease
- Nephrotic syndrome
- Severe hypercalcaemia (used in conjunction with intravenous fluids).

Contraindications

- Renal failure with anuria.

Common side effects

The fluid and electrolyte abnormalities are similar to those of thiazide diuretics (see above), with the following exceptions:

- Hypercalcaemia does not occur.
- Metabolic effects are less common.

Specific adverse effects of loop diuretics include ototoxicity and nephrotoxicity.

Significant interactions

For significant interactions of loop diuretics, see Table 3.3.

Potassium-sparing diuretics and aldosterone antagonists

Mechanism of action (Figure 3.2)

Spironolactone acts as an aldosterone antagonist at the collecting ducts. Amiloride and triamterene interact with luminal membrane sodium channels. All three drugs produce an increase in sodium clearance and a decrease in K^+ and H^+ excretion. Spironolactone has a slow onset and offset of action lasting up to 72 hours, whereas triamterene and amiloride act for 12–24 hours.

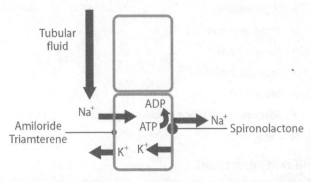

Figure 3.2 Mechanism of action of potassium-sparing diuretics on the distal tubules and collecting ducts.

Examples

- Amiloride
- Triamterene
- Spironolactone.

Example prescription

SPIRONOLACTONE 100 mg p.o. o.d.

Indications

- Traditionally used to prevent the hypokalaemia caused by thiazide and loop diuretics (their use in this regard is declining because of increasing prescribing of other drugs that cause potassium retention, eg angiotensin-converting enzyme [ACE] inhibitors and angiotensin-II receptor antagonists)

- Heart failure
- Chronic liver disease.

Contraindications
- Hyperkalaemia
- Renal failure.

Common side effects
- Hyperkalaemia
- Hyponatraemia
- Breast tenderness*
- Gynaecomastia*
- Testicular atrophy*
- Impotence*
- Mild androgenic effects in women, eg hirsutism*.

*Spironolactone

Significant interactions
Hyperkalaemia occurs most commonly in patients with impaired renal function and those receiving potassium supplements, ACE inhibitors, angiotensin II receptor antagonists, non-steroidal anti-inflammatory drugs or β blockers.

Beta blockers

Mechanism of action
Beta blockers are competitive antagonists at β adrenoceptors. They reduce oxygen demand by decreasing heart rate, blood pressure and myocardial contractility. Beta blockers are therefore the drugs of first choice in the treatment of angina pectoris. They also reduce infarct size after a myocardial infarction and decrease mortality and reinfarction. The mechanisms responsible for the blood pressure-lowering effects of beta blockers are unknown, but inhibition of renin release by the kidney and resetting of the baroreceptors are the most widely accepted theories. More recently, they have been shown to decrease mortality and reduce hospital admissions in patients with congestive cardiac failure. Blockade of the β receptors is also effective in reducing tremor and palpitations in situational anxiety and thyrotoxicosis.

Drug	Selectivity	Lipid solubility	Local anaesthetic	Partial agonist activity
Atenolol	β_1	Low	None	None
Bisoprolol	β_1	Low	None	None
Carvedilol	β_1, β_2	—	—	None
Pindolol	β_1, β_2	Moderate	Yes	Yes
Propranolol	β_1, β_2	High	Yes	None
Timolol	β_1, β_2	Moderate	None	None

Table 3.4 Properties of commonly used β blockers

These drugs are subclassified on the basis of selectivity, lipid solubility, local anaesthetic properties and partial agonist activity (Table 3.4). Some have additional vasodilator and α-blocking activity.

Receptor selectivity

Several β blockers (bisoprolol, atenolol, metoprolol) have greater activity at the β_1 receptor than at the β_2 receptor. Propranolol and sotalol are drugs that are non-selective and have important effects at the β_2 receptor. Selective β blockers cause less bronchoconstriction and less impaired muscle blood flow.

Partial agonist activity

Pindolol and acebutolol do not achieve full antagonist activity at the β receptor. They have less effect on the resting heart rate than other β blockers but have no clear clinical advantages.

Local anaesthetic activity

Propranolol has additional effects on inhibiting the sodium channel in cardiac muscle and peripheral sensory nerves. No clear advantage has been identified for this property, but propranolol is associated with increased cardiotoxicity in overdose and cannot be used to treat glaucoma because it acts as an anaesthetic and can increase the risk of corneal ulceration.

Lipid solubility

Lipid-soluble β blockers such as propranolol demonstrate first-pass hepatic metabolism, greater plasma concentration variability, shorter half-lives and a higher incidence of disturbed sleep. Water-soluble drugs such as atenolol and sotalol undergo less hepatic metabolism, have longer elimination half-lives and cause less sleep disturbance.

Additional properties

Labetalol and carvedilol have additional α-blocking or vasodilator properties, and sotalol has type III anti-arrhythmic activity.

Examples

- Atenolol
- Bisoprolol
- Metoprolol
- Sotalol
- Carvedilol
- Pindolol
- Propranolol
- Timolol.

Example prescription

BISOPROLOL 2.5 mg p.o. o.d.

Indications

Beta blockers are used in a wide variety of clinical situations (Table 3.5).

Contraindications

For contraindications, see Table 3.6.

Clinical condition	Preferred agents	Effect
Hypertension	Cardioselective eg atenolol, bisoprolol	Reduced renin release Baroreceptor adjustment to reduced cardiac output and heart rate
Angina pectoris	Cardioselective agents eg atenolol, bisoprolol Avoid drugs with partial agonist activity	Reduced oxygen demand as a result of reduced heart rate, reduced blood pressure and myocardial contractility
Congestive heart failure	Bisoprolol Carvedilol Metoprolol	Mechanism unclear
Post-myocardial infarction	Selective and non-selective	Possibly reduced risk of arrhythmia?
Migraine	Propranolol	Mechanism unclear
Glaucoma	Timolol	Reduced secretion of aqueous humour

Table 3.5 Clinical uses of β blockers

Condition	Absolute	Relative
Cardiac	Severe bradycardia Heart block Left ventricular failure	? Prinzmetal's angina Patient already receiving drugs that depress sinoatrial or atrioventricular nodes (verapamil, diltiazem, digoxin, anti-arrhythmic drugs)
Pulmonary	Severe asthma	Mild asthma or obstructive airway disease
CNS	Severe depression	Visual hallucinations Vivid dreams Fatigue
Peripheral vascular	Severe peripheral vascular disease – gangrene, necrosis, rest pain	Cold extremities Raynaud's phenomenon Absent pulses
Diabetes	—	Avoid non-selective agents in patients prone to hypoglycaemia
Pregnancy	—	Avoid non-selective agents in favour of labetalol and atenolol

Table 3.6 Contraindications to the use of β blockers

Common side effects

- Bradycardia
- Heart block
- Congestive heart failure (even though this can be used in its treatment)
- Hypotension
- Bronchoconstriction in patients with asthma
- Mask the clinical features of hypoglycaemia (non-selective β blockers)
- Vivid dreams and sleep disturbance (lipid-soluble drugs)
- Worsening of Raynaud's phenomenon
- Cold extremities
- Intermittent claudication.

Significant interactions

The combination of β blockers with class I anti-arrhythmic drugs, anaesthetics and rate-limiting calcium channel blockers can cause severe cardiac depression. Verapamil, diltiazem and cardiac glycosides further depress atrioventricular (AV) conduction and can cause bradycardia and heart block. Sudden increases in heart rate and blood pressure can occur after drug withdrawal, sometimes accompanied by prolonged chest pain. Rebound hypertension is more common if clonidine is co-administered, probably a result of upregulation of the β receptors. The combination with thiazide diuretics increases the risk of developing diabetes.

Calcium channel-blocking drugs

Mechanism of action

Calcium channel blockers work at a cellular level by blocking the voltage-gated L-type calcium channels in cardiac and vascular smooth muscle. As a result they induce vasodilation and to a lesser degree relax the smooth muscle of the uterus, bronchi and gastrointestinal tract.

Calcium channel blockers are subdivided into 'rate-limiting' and 'non-rate-limiting' types:

- Rate-limiting (associated with reduced heart rate, decreased cardiac conduction and contraction): verapamil and diltiazem

- Non-rate-limiting (dihydropyridine group that tends to have greater effects on blood vessels and secondary increases in heart rate, especially if rapid-acting): nifedipine and amlodipine.

The rate and contractility of the heart are reduced by verapamil and diltiazem. These rate-limiting calcium channel blockers also block conduction in the AV node and are sometimes used to treat nodal tachycardias. The dihydropyridine calcium channel blockers produce greater vasodilatation with resulting sympathetic activation and increased heart rate. All calcium channel blockers reduce blood pressure.

Example prescription

AMLODIPINE 5 mg p.o. o.d.

Indications

- Prophylactic therapy in stable and unstable angina
- Hypertension
- Cluster headaches
- Raynaud's disease.

Contraindications

- Poor cardiac output, eg left ventricular failure, significant aortic stenosis
- Bradycardia and heart block (for rate-limiting agents).

Common side effects

- Flushing
- Tachycardia
- Hypotension
- Peripheral oedema
- Constipation (more common with diltiazem and verapamil)
- Congestive heart failure (more common with diltiazem and verapamil)
- Depression of the sinoatrial (SA) and AV nodes (more common with diltiazem and verapamil).

Significant interactions

The rate-limiting calcium channel blockers increase the risk of severe bradycardia and heart block when combined with β blockers.

> **Don't forget**
>
> **Never prescribe a 'rate-limiting' calcium channel blocker with a β blocker.**

Alpha blockers

Mechanism of action (Figure 3.3)

These drugs are antagonists at the α-adrenoceptor. The main mode of action is to reduce peripheral resistance by dilating arterioles. Selective α_1 blockers block the postsynaptic α_1-receptor and do not facilitate the release of noradrenaline (norepinephrine) from the sympathetic nerve endings. As a result they are more effective in reducing blood pressure than non-selective agents and do not induce reflex tachycardia.

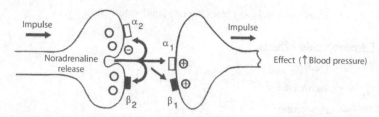

Figure 3.3 Sympathetic nerve ending sharing α and β receptors.

Examples

- Prazosin
- Doxazosin.

Example prescription

DOXAZOSIN 4 mg p.o. o.d.

Indications

- Hypertension
- To improve urinary flow in patients with prostatic obstruction.

Contraindications

Not recommended in some patients with heart failure.

Common side effects

- First-dose hypotension with prazosin (uncommon with doxazosin)
- Urinary incontinence (particularly in postmenopausal women with pelvic floor instability).

Significant interactions

None.

Angiotensin-converting enzyme inhibitors

Mechanism of action (Figure 3.4)

ACE inhibitors block the conversion of the inactive decapeptide, angiotensin I, to the active vasoconstrictor octapeptide, angiotensin II. Reductions in the concentrations of angiotensin II produce a decrease in circulating aldosterone, with associated sodium loss and potassium retention. ACE inhibitors also prevent the breakdown of kinins, locally formed vasoactive peptides, which dilate blood vessels and stimulate the synthesis of vasodilatory prostaglandins.

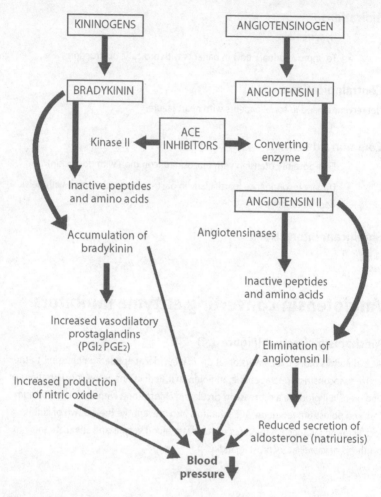

Figure 3.4 Mechanism of action of ACE inhibitors.

ACE inhibitors exert their principal antihypertensive effects by reducing vascular tone in resistance vessels and large arteries. Unlike most other peripheral vasodilators, ACE inhibitors do not produce reflex changes in heart rate, which may be related to reduced sympathetic or increased parasympathetic activity. In hypertensive patients, cardiac output remains unchanged, and for most patients renal perfusion is slightly improved or unaffected. In renal artery stenosis, progressive increases in efferent glomerular arterial tone occur to compensate for reduced renal perfusion. This is largely achieved by increased angiotensin II concentrations. In bilateral renal artery stenosis or stenosis in a solitary kidney, ACE inhibitors can cause acute renal failure by blocking this compensatory mechanism. Deterioration in renal function after ACE inhibition is, however, most commonly seen in patients with heart failure and generalised atherosclerosis who are hypotensive and volume depleted as a result of diuretic therapy.

Examples

- Captopril
- Enalapril
- Lisinopril
- Ramipril
- Perindopril
- Trandolapril.

Example prescription

RAMIPRIL 2.5 mg p.o. o.d.

Indications

- Reduced left ventricular systolic function (in asymptomatic patients ACE inhibitors prevent the development of symptomatic heart failure, and in those with heart failure they reduce mortality and delay further deterioration in ventricular systolic function)
- Hypertension
- After a myocardial infarction (MI) (the main benefit after an MI appears to be related to improved systolic function in patients with impaired cardiac output)
- High cardiovascular risk groups (largely related to decreases in blood pressure)
- Renoprotective effects in patients with diabetes and those with renal hypertension.

Contraindications

Known hypersensitivity, renal artery stenosis or pregnancy.

Common side effects

- Non-productive cough
- Hypotension, particularly after the first dose
- Acute renal insufficiency, especially with bilateral renal artery stenosis
- Hyperkalaemia
- Angioedema.

Significant interactions

Potassium-sparing diuretics and angiotensin-II receptor antagonists increase the risk of hyperkalaemia in patients with renal impairment. Non-steroidal anti-inflammatory drugs (NSAIDs) reduce the antihypertensive effect and blunt the effects of ACE inhibitors in congestive heart failure.

Angiotensin-II receptor antagonists

Mechanism of action (Figure 3.5)

Angiotensin-II receptor antagonists bind competitively and non-competitively to the angiotensin AT_1 receptor, blocking the effects of angiotensin II at that receptor. This results in relaxation of vascular smooth muscle, reduced aldosterone release and decreased cell growth and proliferation.

Angiotensin receptor antagonists produce effects similar to those of ACE inhibitors but, because they do not affect the kinin–prostaglandin system, they do not cause cough.

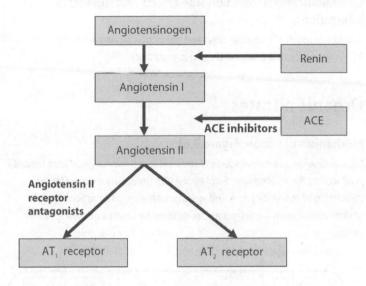

Figure 3.5 Antihypertensive drugs that inhibit the renin–angiotensin system.

Examples

- Losartan
- Candesartan
- Irbesartan
- Valsartan.

Example prescription

LOSARTAN 50 mg p.o. o.d.

Indications

The main indication for angiotensin-II receptor antagonists is for treating patients who develop an ACE inhibitor induced cough. A losartan-based antihypertensive treatment is associated with a better outcome than a regimen based on atenolol. They are not superior to ACE inhibitors in heart failure or after an MI, but have a better evidence base in patients with type 2 diabetes and renal impairment.

Contraindications, common side effects and significant interactions

Apart from cough, the adverse effect and interaction profiles are similar to those of ACE inhibitors; both are contraindicated in pregnancy.

Organic nitrates

Mechanism of action (Figure 3.6)

Nitrates provide an external source of nitric oxide, a powerful vasodilator naturally produced by the endothelium. Sulphhydryl (SH) groups are required for the stimulation of guanylyl cyclase, and vascular tolerance to the action of organic nitrates occurs when the SH groups are oxidised by excess exposure to nitrate groups.

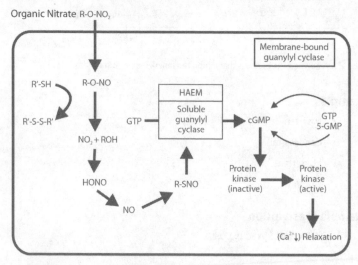

Figure 3.6 Proposed cellular actions of organic nitrates. PDE, phosphodiesterase.

Nitrates relax all vascular smooth muscle but they have greater venous than arterial effects. In angina, by causing venodilatation they reduce venous pressure and left ventricular volume, and by dilating resistance vessels they decrease systemic blood pressure. The overall effect is reduced ventricular wall tension and myocardial oxygen demand. These effects are also beneficial in heart failure. In reducing left ventricular filling pressure and volume, these drugs can produce symptomatic relief in acute pulmonary oedema caused by left heart failure.

Examples

- Sublingual glyceryl trinitrate
- Oral isosorbide mononitrate
- Oral isosorbide dinitrate
- Buccal glyceryl trinitrate
- Transdermal glyceryl trinitrate
- Intravenous glyceryl trinitrate
- Intravenous isosorbide dinitrate.

Glyceryl trinitrate has low oral bioavailability because of extensive hepatic first-pass metabolism. If swallowed, therefore, the drug has little or no clinical activity. It is also highly lipid soluble and well absorbed through the skin and buccal mucosa. Transdermal, buccal and sublingual preparations make use of this property. As both transdermal and intravenous administration result in continuous exposure of the drug to the receptor, tolerance is most common with these forms of delivery.

Example prescriptions

GLYCERYL TRINITRATE 800µg s.l. p.r.n.

ISOSORBIDE MONONITRATE 20mg p.o. b.d.

Indications

- Angina pectoris (glyceryl trinitrate administered sublingually is useful as a prophylactic and a diagnostic agent, as well as being useful in the treatment of an acute attack. Oral nitrates are useful for prophylaxis, but require a 6- to 8-hour 'nitrate-free interval' to prevent nitrate tolerance. Intravenous nitrates are useful in severe unstable angina but transdermal nitrates are of little clinical value)
- Acute pulmonary oedema
- Heart failure (organic nitrates have a limited role in the treatment of heart failure. They are used to improve symptoms and reduce mortality when ACE inhibitors and/or β blockers are contraindicated, and intravenously with loop diuretics in severe refractory left ventricular failure).

Contraindications

Hypotension and left ventricular outflow obstruction (ie significant aortic stenosis or hypertrophic obstructive cardiomyopathy).

Common side effects

- Hypotension
- Tachycardia
- Headache.

Significant interactions

None.

All these effects are greater when nitrates are administered together with sildenafil (Viagra®), alcohol or calcium channel blockers.

Inotropes

Drugs with inotropic activity produce their effect by increasing the availability of intracellular free calcium to the contractile proteins within the myocardium. Increased sensitivity to calcium may also play a role. Three classes of inotropes are commonly used.

Cardiac glycosides

Mechanism of action (Figure 3.7)

The principal cellular action of the cardiac glycosides is inhibition of the enzyme Na^+/K^+ ATPase on the myocardial cell membrane. This results in an increase in intracellular sodium, which in turn reduces the release of calcium from the cell by activation of the Na^+/Ca^{2+} exchanger. Intracellular calcium levels rise by this and other mechanisms.

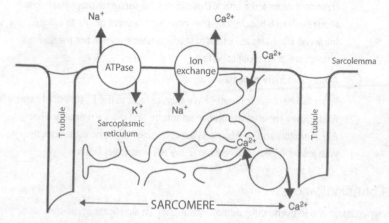

Figure 3.7 Possible sites of action of the cardiac glycosides.

These drugs exert a number of electrophysiological effects directly on the heart or indirectly by interacting with the autonomic nervous system. The myocardial action potential is reduced and the conducting system, particularly at the AV node, becomes refractory to incoming impulses. A fall in heart rate is largely the result of reduced sympathetic and increased parasympathetic effects. At high concentrations, however, increased sympathetic effects are observed, which are largely responsible for the drug's pro-arrhythmic effects.

In heart failure the main beneficial effects of the cardiac glycosides are a reduction of ventricular rate in atrial fibrillation and a small inotropic effect in patients with sinus rhythm. The clinical benefits reported in patients with sinus rhythm are small but it is the only inotrope for which long-term use is not associated with increased mortality.

Digoxin and digitoxin have long half-lives mainly as a result of their large apparent volumes of distribution. It has been traditional to employ a loading dose in order to achieve therapeutic plasma concentrations more rapidly, but recent evidence suggests that this is rarely necessary. Digoxin, the glycoside that is exclusively used in the UK, is largely eliminated by the kidney and, because of its narrow therapeutic index, needs to be adjusted for changes in renal function. Digitoxin undergoes extensive metabolism and reduction of the dose is less important in patients with renal impairment.

Box 3.1 Factors increasing sensitivity to cardiac glycosides

Underlying disease	Electrolyte disorders
Cor pulmonale	Hypokalaemia
Hypothyroidism	Hypomagnesaemia
Chronic rheumatic or viral carditis	Hypercalcaemia
Acute MI	

Examples

- Digoxin
- Digitoxin.

Example prescription

DIGOXIN 250 micrograms p.o. o.d.

Indications

- Heart failure
- Fast atrial fibrillation.

Contraindications

- Second- or third-degree AV block
- Wolff–Parkinson–White syndrome
- Ventricular tachycardia
- Hypertrophic obstructive cardiomyopathy.

Common side effects

- Anorexia
- Nausea
- Confusion
- Diarrhoea
- Visual disturbances: yellow–green vision, halos around objects and blurred images
- Almost any dysrhythmia can occur in patients with digoxin toxicity (Figure 3.8). The most common are ventricular ectopics, including bigeminal rhythm, AV junctional escape rhythms, atrial tachycardia with AV block, ventricular tachycardia and sinus arrest. Fast atrial fibrillation is more likely to be the result of inadequate treatment rather than toxicity. All degrees of heart block can occur.

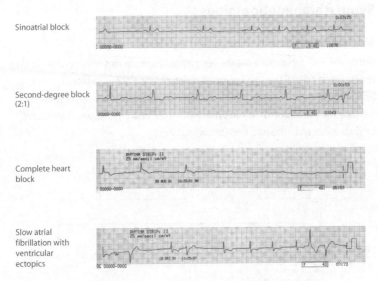

Sinoatrial block

Second-degree block (2:1)

Complete heart block

Slow atrial fibrillation with ventricular ectopics

Figure 3.8 A selection of common rhythm disturbances resulting from digoxin toxicity.

Significant interactions

The main pharmacodynamic interactions with digoxin and digitoxin include those with the loop and thiazide diuretics that predispose to hypokalaemia, and the combination with drugs that impair cardiac conduction – class I and III anti-arrhythmics, β blockers and rate-limiting calcium channel blockers. Important pharmacokinetic interactions are listed inTable 3.7.

Drug	Average increase in steady-state plasma digoxin concentrations (%)
Amiodarone	70–100
Propafenone	25–35
Quinidine	100
Spironolactone	20
Verapamil	50–100

Table 3.7 Some important cardiovascular drugs which increase the serum digoxin concentration

Sympathomimetic amines

Mechanism of action (Figure 3.9)

Dopamine and dobutamine are the sympathomimetic amines most commonly used to treat heart failure. They act principally by stimulating adrenoceptors. Adrenoceptors are G-protein-coupled receptors that activate adenylyl cyclase and increase the conversion of ATP to cyclic AMP. In the heart this results in increased calcium influx and increased force of contraction.

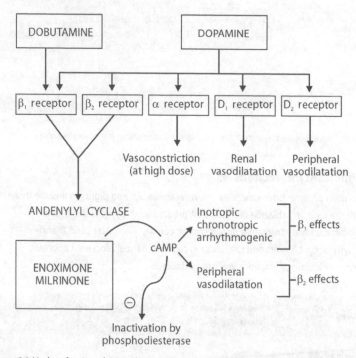

Figure 3.9 Modes of action of sympathomimetic amines and phosphodiesterase inhibitors.

Examples

- Dopamine
- Dobutamine.

Example prescription

DOBUTAMINE 250 micrograms per minute by continuous i.v. infusion

Indications

- Severe heart failure
- Cardiogenic shock after an acute MI or drug overdose.

Contraindication

- Tachycardia.

Common side effects

- Arrhythmias
- Sudden death.

Tolerance is a problem and infusions should not be administered for more than 72 hours. Long-term use is associated with increased mortality.

Significant interactions

- Risks of autonomic instability when administered with other drugs affecting the autonomic nervous system

Phosphodiesterase inhibitors

Mechanism of action (Figure 3.9)

Inhibition of phosphodiesterase results in increased intracellular cyclic AMP in cardiac muscle, with subsequent phosphorylation of cellular proteins by cAMP-dependent protein kinase. The two main effects of phosphodiesterase inhibitors are the stimulation of the force of myocardial cells and relaxation of arteriolar smooth muscle. They are sometimes known as 'inodilators'.

Examples

- Milrinone
- Enoximone.

Example prescription

MILRINONE 50 micrograms per minute by continuous i.v. infusion

Indication

- Short-term treatment of severe heart failure unresponsive to other therapies.

Common side effects

- Tachycardia
- Arrhythmias
- Hypotension.

Thrombolytics

Mechanism of action (Figure 3.10)

Thrombolytic agents catalyse the activation of the inactive precursor plasminogen to plasmin, which is the normal fibrinolytic enzyme. By splitting fibrin into fragments, plasmin promotes the dissolution of thrombus.

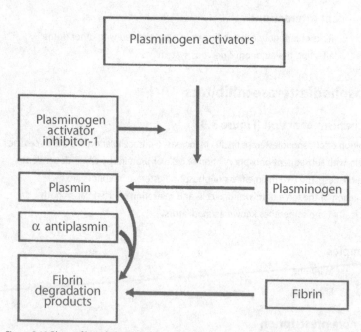

Figure 3.10 Plasma fibrinolytic system.

The thrombolytic agents produce a rapid and a short duration of effect. The thrombin time usually returns to less than twice the normal value within a few hours of administration, but the prothrombin time can be prolonged for up to 24 hours as a result of reduced fibrinogen and other clotting factors. Table 3.8 shows some of the advantages and disadvantages of commonly available agents.

Drug	Advantages	Disadvantages
Streptokinase	Clinically proved value Relatively inexpensive	Antigenic Occasional allergic reaction Hypotension
Anistreplase	Clinically proved value Rapid effect with prolonged action	Antigenic Occasional allergic reaction Moderately expensive
Alteplase	Clinically proved value Non-antigenic Highly clot selective	Simultaneous heparin therapy required Short half-life Very expensive

Table 3.8 Advantages and disadvantages of three commonly available thrombolytic agents

Examples

- Streptokinase
- Anistreplase
- Alteplase
- Reteplase.

Example prescription

RETEPLASE 10 units i.v. stat

Followed by:

RETEPLASE 10 units i.v. 30 minutes later

Indications

- Acute coronary artery thrombosis (best results are achieved if the drug is administered intravenously within 4 hours of the onset. Later administration is associated with reduced efficacy and increased risk of bleeding)
- Large or multiple pulmonary emboli.

Contraindications

- Recent haemorrhage (including intracerebral haemorrhage)
- Recent trauma (including surgery)
- Defective coagulation
- Aortic dissection
- Peptic ulceration
- Severe hypertension
- Oesophageal varices.

Common side effects

- Bleeding, including intracerebral haemorrhage
- Transient hypotension
- Arrhythmias
- Allergic reactions (these occur in about 12% of patients after streptokinase treatment and are most commonly observed in patients who are re-exposed within a period of 6 months; other thrombolytic drugs are therefore preferred for second or subsequent exposure).

Significant interactions

Anticoagulant and antiplatelet drugs, which increase the risk of bleeding.

Anti-arrhythmic drugs

These drugs are usually classified as shown in Figure 3.11.

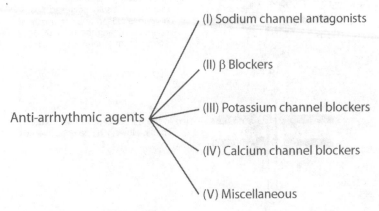

Figure 3.11 Classification of anti-arrhythmic agents.

Class I (sodium channel antagonists)

These are subclassified into three types as shown in Table 3.9.

IA	IB	IC
Quinidine Procainamide Disopyramide	Lidocaine Mexiletine Phenytoin	Flecainide Propafenone

Table 3.9 Types of class I anti-arrhythmic drugs

Mechanism of action (Figure 3.12)

As local anaesthetics, all class I drugs slow or block conduction (especially in depolarised cells) and slow or abolish abnormal pacemaker activity, which is related to the sodium channel. At a cellular level, these drugs bind to their receptors more readily when the sodium channel is open or inactivated than when it is fully repolarised. As abnormal tissue has more cells in the open or inactivated state, sodium channel blockers have a greater effect on abnormal conducting tissue. Table 3.10 summarises the cellular and conduction effects of the class I drugs.

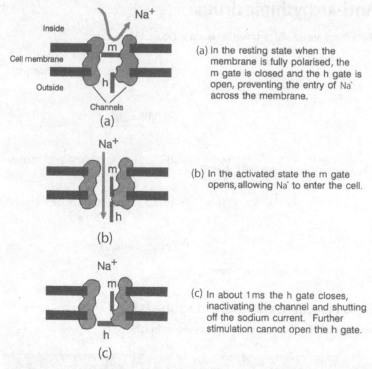

(a) In the resting state when the membrane is fully polarised, the m gate is closed and the h gate is open, preventing the entry of Na⁺ across the membrane.

(b) In the activated state the m gate opens, allowing Na⁺ to enter the cell.

(c) In about 1 ms the h gate closes, inactivating the channel and shutting off the sodium current. Further stimulation cannot open the h gate.

Figure 3.12 Schematic diagrams of the cardiac sodium channel during resting (a), activated (b) and inactivated (c) stages.

Examples

See Table 3.9.

Class	Cellular action	Main sites of action	Effects on the ECG
IA	Block 1_{Na} and 1_{Kr}	Atria Purkinje fibres Ventricular cells	QRS and Q–T lengthening
IB	Block 1_{Na}	Purkinje fibres Ventricular cells	Little effect at therapeutic doses
IC	Block 1_{Na}	Atria Ventricular cells	QRS widening

Table 3.10 Cellular and conduction effects of class I anti-arrhythmics

Example prescription

FLECAINIDE 50 mg p.o. t.i.d.

Indications

- Atrial arrhythmias
- Ventricular arrhythmias.

The use of these agents has declined because they also have pro-arrhythmic effects and can increase sudden death. The use of class I anti-arrhythmic agents is therefore usually limited to the treatment of serious refractory and symptomatic rhythm disturbance. Lidocaine is of no value in acute MI unless severe ventricular arrhythmias are present.

Common side effects

Class IA

All have anti-muscarinic effects, especially disopyramide, and can cause heart failure. All are pro-arrhythmic. Quinidine causes adverse effects associated with quinine:

- Headache
- Vertigo
- Tinnitus
- Gastrointestinal symptoms
- Thrombocytopenia.

Class IB

- Confusion
- Disorientation
- Convulsions.

Class IC

- Pro-arrhythmic
- Sudden death.

Significant interactions

Quinidine increases the plasma concentrations of digoxin and, therefore, the risk of digoxin toxicity. It also increases the anticoagulant effects of warfarin. Additive effects on cardiac conduction and contraction are seen with β blockers, 'rate-limiting' calcium channel blockers and with drugs that increase the Q–T interval.

Class II (β blockers)

See page 52 for details.

Class III (potassium channel blockers)

Box 3.2 D-Sotalol and bretylium

D-Sotalol and bretylium are true class III anti-arrhythmic agents and block the 1_{Kr} potassium channels. Their principal effects are lengthening of the cardiac action potential and prolongation of the Q–T interval on the electrocardiogram (ECG). However, they are almost never used in the UK and the preference is for amiodarone.

Amiodarone

Mechanism of action

Amiodarone has class I as well as III and weak class II and IV effects. It blocks sodium and calcium channels as well as potassium channels, and has weak β-adrenoceptor blocking activity.

As a result of its multiple anti-arrhythmic effects, amiodarone slows the sinus rate and AV conduction and lengthens the QRS and Q–T duration on the ECG. Atrial, AV and ventricular refractory periods are increased. The pro-arrhythmic effects of amiodarone are less than with most other orally active anti-arrhythmic agents. Amiodarone also dilates resistance and coronary arteries and sometimes causes hypotension at high doses.

Amiodarone has a very large apparent volume of distribution and an elimination half-life that ranges from 26 to 107 days during chronic administration. As a result, the onset of action is delayed and steady-state concentrations are not achieved for several months. A loading dose is required to achieve early therapeutic concentrations.

Example prescription

AMIODARONE 200 mg p.o. o.d.

Indications

- Life-threatening ventricular arrhythmias
- Recurrent cardiac arrest
- Atrial fibrillation
- Atrial flutter
- Paroxysmal supraventricular tachycardia.

Contraindications

- Bradycardia
- SA heart block
- Thyroid disease
- Iodine hypersensitivity
- Pregnancy.

Common side effects

- Corneal deposits
- Hyper- or hypothyroidism
- Liver function abnormalities
- Peripheral neuropathy
- Photosensitivity
- Slate-grey skin pigmentation
- Pulmonary fibrosis.

Significant interactions

Amiodarone increases the anticoagulant effect of warfarin and doubles the steady-state plasma concentrations of digoxin. Problems are likely to occur if amiodarone is combined with other drugs that increase the Q–T interval or depress nodal activity.

Class IV (calcium channel blockers)

See page 56 for details.

Class V (miscellaneous)

Adenosine

When administered as an intravenous bolus, adenosine slows conduction in the AV node, probably by hyperpolarising this tissue via the 1_{Kr} channel. It is extremely effective in abolishing AV nodal arrhythmias and is widely used in accident and emergency departments for this purpose. Main adverse effects include short-lived flushing, hypotension, chest pain and dyspnoea.

Magnesium and sodium

Magnesium is useful in the treatment of torsade de pointes ventricular tachycardia, and sodium bicarbonate is useful for arrhythmias induced by class I anti-arrhythmic drugs and tricyclic antidepressant overdoses.

Lipid-lowering agents

Hydroxymethylglutaryl coenzyme A reductase inhibitors (statins)

Mechanism of action (Figure 3.13)

Statins competitively inhibit mevalonate synthesis by hydroxymethylglutaryl coenzyme A (HMG-CoA) reductase, a process essential for cholesterol biosynthesis in the liver. The liver compensates by increasing the number of low-density lipoprotein (LDL) receptors. As a result, the clearance of very-low-density lipoprotein (VLDL) remnants and LDL from the blood increases.

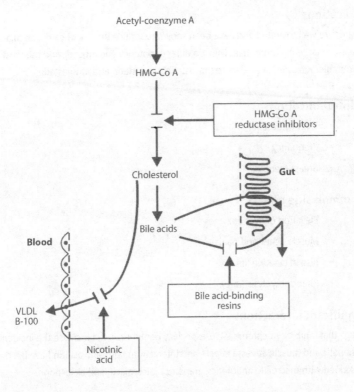

Figure 3.13 Main sites of action of HMG-CoA reductase inhibitors, bile acid-binding resins and nicotinic acid.

Examples

- Pravastatin
- Simvastatin
- Atorvastatin.

Example prescription

PRAVASTATIN 10 mg p.o o.d.

Indications

Statins are well tolerated and have been shown to reduce the risk of cardiovascular disease in large outcome trials. They do differ in potency and efficacy, and the most favourable outcome data relate to pravastatin, simvastatin and atorvastatin.

Contraindications

- Liver disease
- Pregnancy
- Breast-feeding.

Common side effects

- Elevation of liver enzymes
- Muscle aches and pains
- Rise in creatine kinase
- Rhabdomyolysis (rare).

Significant interactions

Drugs that inhibit cytochrome P450, especially gemfibrozil, can increase the incidence of hepatic and muscle adverse effects, and interactions with simvastatin have been described with macrolide antibiotics, grapefruit juice, niacin and ciclosporin.

Fibric acid derivatives (fibrates)

Mechanism of action (Figure 3.14)

Fibrates act as ligands for peroxisome proliferator-activated receptor-α (PPAR-α), a receptor that regulates the transcription of genes involved in lipid metabolism. The overall effect is to increase lipoprotein lipase and the clearance of triglyceride-rich lipoproteins. LDL-cholesterol is reduced and HDL-cholesterol is increased.

Overall, the clinical outcome data for fibrates have been disappointing. The reduction in LDL-cholesterol is modest and statins are preferred for the prevention of cardiovascular disease.

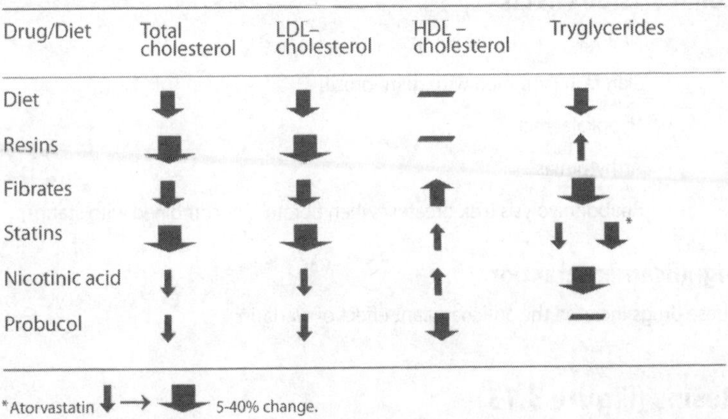

Drug/Diet	Total cholesterol	LDL–cholesterol	HDL –cholesterol	Tryglycerides
Diet	⬇	⬇	—	⬇
Resins	⬇	⬇	—	↑
Fibrates	⬇	⬇	⬆	⬇
Statins	⬇	⬇	↑	↓ ⬇*
Nicotinic acid	↓	↓	↑	⬇
Probucol	↓	↓	⬇	—

*Atorvastatin ↓ ⟶ ⬇ 5-40% change.

Figure 3.14 Effects of drugs (with diet) on plasma lipid profiles in patients with coronary heart disease or mild hypercholesterolaemia for 1 year.

Examples

- Fenofibrate
- Bezafibrate.

Example prescription

FENOFIBRATE 200 mg p.o. o.d.

Indications

Fibrates are frequently used to treat mixed hyperlipidaemia and are often combined with statins. In this condition, which is common in patients with diabetes, the triglycerides are elevated and HDL-cholesterol is reduced.

Contraindications

- Severe renal or liver disease
- Pregnancy
- Breast-feeding.

Common side effects

- Nausea
- Skin rash (common with gemfibrozil)
- Hypokalaemia
- Arrhythmias
- Rhabdomyolysis (risk greatest when fibrates are combined with statins).

Significant interactions

These drugs increase the anticoagulant effect of warfarin.

Resins (Figure 3.13)

Bile acid-binding resins (colestyramine and colestipol) bind bile acids and related steroids in the intestine. They are occasionally used to reduce cholesterol in severe hypercholesterolaemia, but their use is limited by a very high incidence of bloating, constipation and disturbances of taste. Resins prevent the absorption of other drugs and fat-soluble vitamins.

Nicotinic acid (Figure 3.13)

Niacin has been used for many years in the USA as a lipid-lowering agent and it is the most effective drug for increasing HDLs and lowering triglycerides. Favourable clinical outcome data are available for patients with mixed hyperlipidaemia and low HDLs but its use is limited by a high incidence of flushing, nausea and abdominal discomfort. Hyperuricaemia, impaired carbohydrate tolerance and liver impairment can also occur.

Management of acute MI

- Make the patient as comfortable as possible.
- Give high-flow oxygen (60–100%) unless the patient has evidence of CO_2 retention.
- Give pain relief using an opiate slowly intravenously – 2.5–5.0 mg diamorphine, often combined with metoclopramide to reduce the risk of vomiting.

- Administer 150–300 mg aspirin.
- If there are no contraindications give a thrombolytic agent as soon as possible if the ECG demonstrates ST-segment elevation and/or new left bundle branch block.
- If thrombolytics are given, heparin should be given for at least 24 hours to help prevent re-thrombosis.
- Intravenous isosorbide dinitrate can be used to relieve ischaemic pain.
- Treat associated rhythm disturbances:
  - atrial fibrillation: 500 micrograms to 1 mg digoxin orally unless the patient cannot swallow
  - sinus bradycardia: atropine 600 micrograms to 1.2 mg
  - ventricular tachycardia: consider lidocaine intravenously and DC shock
  - heart block: pacing.

Beta blockers and ACE inhibitors, when administered early after an MI, can limit infarct size and reduce the risk of subsequent heart failure.

Long-term management

- 75 mg aspirin reduces the risk of re-infarction.
- Beta blockers reduce the risk of arrhythmias and prevent sudden death.
- ACE inhibitors prevent the development of heart failure in patients with left ventricular dysfunction.
- Statins reduce overall cardiovascular risk.

Management of acute left ventricular failure

- Sit the patient upright.
- Give high-flow oxygen (60–100%) unless the patient has evidence of CO_2 retention.
- Administer a loop diuretic, eg furosemide 20–80 mg intravenously.
- Give an opiate slowly intravenously: 2.5–5.0 mg diamorphine/morphine. Opiates are commonly combined with antiemetics to reduce the risk of

vomiting. Watch for and treat respiratory depressant effects.

- Treat associated rhythm disturbances:

    - atrial fibrillation: 500 micrograms to 1 mg digoxin orally unless the patient cannot swallow

    - sinus bradycardia: atropine 600 micrograms to 1.2 mg

    - ventricular tachycardia: consider lidocaine intravenously and DC shock

    - heart block: pacing.

Most patients will respond to these measures but if the patient remains breathless consider the following:

- Further doses of intravenous furosemide, especially if the patient has significant renal impairment.

- Intravenous isosorbide dinitrate if the systolic blood pressure is > 100 mmHg.

- Intravenous dobutamine if the systolic blood pressure is < 100 mg.

- Venesection.

References

Johnston GD. *Fundamentals of Cardiovascular Pharmacology*. Chichester: John Wiley & Sons, 1999, p 136.

4
Respiratory system

Respiratory system

Asthma and chronic obstructive pulmonary disease

Essential physiology

Asthma is characterised by acute airway obstruction that reverses spontaneously or with therapy, and gives symptoms of wheeze, cough and dyspnoea. Chronic obstructive pulmonary disease (COPD) is also characterised by airflow obstruction but, in contrast to asthma, it is slowly progressive and does not change markedly either spontaneously or in response to treatment. In COPD there is a chronic inflammatory response in the lungs, in response to noxious particles and gases, such as those found in cigarette smoke.

Asthma is primarily an inflammatory disorder, with bronchial hyperreactivity and resultant bronchospasm. Mast cells are distributed throughout the respiratory tract. These cells have receptors for the immunoglobulin IgE. If an antigen to which a person has been sensitised enters the respiratory tract, the complex of mast cell, IgE and antigen triggers degranulation of the mast cell, with release of inflammatory mediators such as histamine. These mediators act on receptors on bronchial smooth muscle cells, causing bronchoconstriction and increased endothelial permeability. The latter causes bronchial mucosal oedema. Other proinflammatory mediators such as prostacyclins, kinins and leukotrienes are released from mast cells via the arachidonic pathway (see page 236).

Respiratory tract smooth muscle is found from the trachea to the terminal bronchioles and is innervated by sympathetic and parasympathetic nerves. Stimulation of β_2 adrenoceptors causes bronchodilatation, whereas vagal stimulation via muscarinic receptors causes bronchial smooth muscle constriction. Beta$_2$ agonists and anticholinergics are therefore used therapeutically as bronchodilators.

Drugs that stabilise mast cells, steroids (which are anti-inflammatory) and leukotriene receptor antagonists are also used in the treatment of asthma.

Routes of drug delivery in respiratory disease

Drugs may be delivered to the lungs by inhalation or by oral or intravenous routes. The choice of route depends on the drug, the disease, the nature of the disease and severity.

Inhaled route

Inhalation is the preferred mode of delivery of many drugs used for respiratory disease. The major advantage of this route is that the drug is delivered directly to the area where it is effective, with a lower risk of systemic side effects, and a more rapid onset of action than when taken orally. However, only a small proportion (around 5–10%) of the inhaled drug reaches the smaller airways.

Inhaled drugs can be delivered by the following means:

- Metered-dose inhaler (MDI): drugs are propelled as an aerosol from a canister with a propellant (now chlorofluorocarbon or CFC free). The patient must coordinate activation of the device with inhalation.

- Breath-activated inhalers: these devices do not require coordination of activation with inhalation, and are therefore particularly effective in patients who have difficulty mastering the technique required for an MDI.

- Dry powder devices. These require the drugs to be formulated as fine powders with a particle size small enough to reach the lower airways.

- Spacer chambers: these are large hollow cylinders that are used in conjunction with an MDI. Fitting of a spacer device (e.g. Volumatic®, Nebuhaler®) to an MDI removes the need to coordinate activation of the inhaler with inhalation. The MDI can be activated into the chamber, and the aerosol is then inhaled from the one-way valve in the spacer device. Use of a spacer device also reduces the oropharyngeal deposition of the drug.

- Nebuliser: a nebuliser converts a solution of a drug into an aerosol for inhalation. Nebulisers can deliver higher doses of drugs than standard inhalers, but still less than 30% of the drug reaches the airways. Nebulisers are used during acute exacerbations of asthma or COPD, or in chronic disease in patients who have not responded to correctly used inhalers with spacer devices. Nebulisers require an air or oxygen flow rate of 6–8 l/minute. In hospital, this is available as piped air or oxygen. This high-flow rate cannot be achieved with oxygen cylinders or oxygen concentrators in the home. An electrical compressor is needed for home nebulisation. Note that nebulisers should be driven by air if the patient has hypercapnia, to prevent worsening of the hypercapnic state.

Oral route

The oral dose of a drug for pulmonary disease is much higher than its inhaled equivalent dose. This means that systemic side effects are much more likely. Where there is a choice of route (eg β agonist or anticholinergic), the inhaled route is always preferred.

Intravenous route

The intravenous route should be reserved for delivery of drugs in severely ill patients who cannot absorb drugs when given orally, or whose bronchospasm is so severe that tidal volume is markedly reduced, making inhaled drug delivery ineffective.

General principles in the treatment of obstructive airways disease

Management regimens for chronic asthma vary, depending on the severity of symptoms. For infrequent mild symptoms, patients commonly require only the occasional use of a bronchodilator (eg two puffs of a 'reliever' such as salbutamol when they feel wheezy). More frequent or persistent symptoms will require regular bronchodilators and, in addition, regular use of a 'preventer' treatment such as twice-daily inhaled corticosteroid (eg beclometasone 100 micrograms). Doses of bronchodilators and inhaled steroids are stepped up and down, depending on the severity of symptoms and response to treatment. The stepwise approach to asthma management is shown in Figure 4.1.

Figure 4.1 Summary of stepwise management in adults

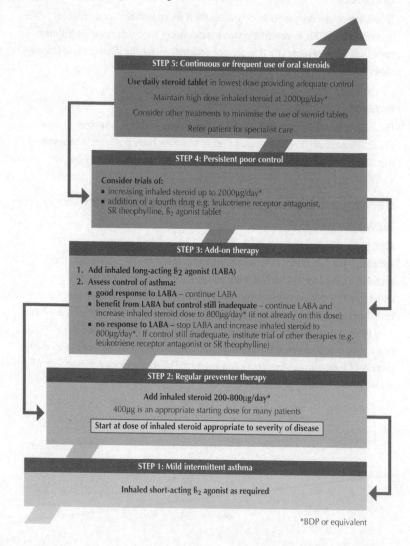

STEP 5: Continuous or frequent use of oral steroids

Use daily steroid tablet in lowest dose providing adequate control

Maintain high dose inhaled steroid at 2000μg/day*

Consider other treatments to minimise the use of steroid tablets

Refer patient for specialist care

STEP 4: Persistent poor control

Consider trials of:
- increasing inhaled steroid up to 2000μg/day*
- addition of a fourth drug e.g. leukotriene receptor antagonist, SR theophylline, ß₂ agonist tablet

STEP 3: Add-on therapy

1. Add inhaled long-acting ß₂ agonist (LABA)
2. Assess control of asthma:
   - good response to LABA – continue LABA
   - benefit from LABA but control still inadequate – continue LABA and increase inhaled steroid dose to 800μg/day* (if not already on this dose)
   - no response to LABA – stop LABA and increase inhaled steroid to 800μg/day*. If control still inadequate, institute trial of other therapies (e.g. leukotriene receptor antagonist or SR theophylline)

STEP 2: Regular preventer therapy

Add inhaled steroid 200-800μg/day*

400μg is an appropriate starting dose for many patients

Start at dose of inhaled steroid appropriate to severity of disease

STEP 1: Mild intermittent asthma

Inhaled short-acting ß₂ agonist as required

*BDP or equivalent

Reproduced with the kind permission of the Scottish Intercollegiate Guidelines Network and British Thoracic Society. Taken from the British Thoracic Society *Thorax*, 2003; **58** (Suppl 1): i1-i92.

In severe chronic airway obstruction, regular long-acting β_2 agonists, theophylline, leukotriene receptor antagonists and mast cell stabilisers may be added to bronchodilator treatment.

The lowest possible dose of inhaled corticosteroid for control of symptoms should be used, in an attempt to minimise side effects. Long-term steroid use (either inhaled or oral) should not be stopped or reduced abruptly, because there will be adrenal suppression and a risk of acute adrenal insufficiency.

For details of treatment regimens for asthma, refer to the British Thoracic Society's *Guidelines on the Management of Asthma* (www.brit-thoracic.org.uk).

For convenience and perhaps improved compliance, combination preparations of some drugs have been developed, eg Combivent® is salbutamol with ipratropium bromide; Symbicort® is budesonide with formoterol.

Bronchodilators

Three groups of bronchodilator drugs are used in asthma and COPD:

- β_2 adrenoceptor agonists
- Anti-muscarinics
- Theophylline.

β_2 Adrenoceptor agonists

Mechanism of action

Selective β_2 agonists are sympathomimetic and cause bronchodilatation by relaxation of bronchial smooth muscle. Short- and long-acting β agonists have been developed.

Examples

Short acting:

- Salbutamol
- Terbutaline
- Fenoterol.

Long acting:

- Salmeterol
- Formoterol.

Example prescriptions

SALBUTAMOL 200 micrograms inhaled p.r.n.

SALBUTAMOL 2.5 mg nebulised q.i.d.

SALMETEROL 50 micrograms inhaled b.d.

Indications

- Asthma
- COPD.

Contraindications

- Hyperthyroidism
- Tachyarrhythmias
- Pregnancy and breast-feeding.

Common side effects

- Tremor
- Tachycardia and palpitations, arrhythmia
- Sleep disturbance
- Muscle cramps
- Hypokalaemia.

Significant interactions

Hypokalaemia when given with corticosteroids, diuretics or theophylline.

Anti-muscarinics

Mechanism of action

These drugs produce bronchodilatation and inhibition of secretions. Unlike atropine, the anti-muscarinics used in COPD do not reduce mucociliary clearance. These drugs compete with acetylcholine for a common binding site on the muscarinic receptor of bronchial smooth muscle. This reduces the bronchoconstrictor effect of vagal tone, which is greater in the airways of patients with COPD.

Examples

- Ipratropium bromide (short acting)
- Tritropium (long acting).

Example prescriptions

IPRATROPIUM BROMIDE 40 micrograms inhaled q.i.d.

TRITROPIUM 18 micrograms inhaled o.d.

Indications

- COPD
- Severe asthma.

Contraindications

- Glaucoma
- Prostatic hypertrophy
- Pregnancy and breast-feeding.

Common side effects

- Dry mouth, pharyngitis
- Nausea
- Headache
- Constipation.

Significant interactions

None.

Theophylline

Mechanism of action

Theophylline is a phosphodiesterase inhibitor. Its administration leads to an increase in intracellular cAMP, which causes bronchodilatation. However, its main effect may be anti-inflammatory. Theophylline inhibits release of mast cell mediators and increases mucociliary clearance. The drug has a narrow therapeutic index and, because of differences in clearance, the dose required to achieve therapeutic blood levels (10–20 mg/l) varies between individuals. Different preparations of theophylline have different bioavailability and, therefore, modified-release preparations must be prescribed by proprietary name.

Example prescriptions

UNIPHYLLIN CONTINUS® 200 mg p.o. b.d.

NUELIN SA® 175 mg p.o. b.d.

Indications

- Acute severe asthma
- Reversible airway obstruction.

Contraindications

- Cardiac disease
- Hyperthyroidism
- Hepatic impairment
- Pregnancy and breast-feeding.

Common side effects

- Palpitations, tachycardia, arrhythmias
- Nausea
- Headaches
- Seizures
- Insomnia.

Significant interactions

- Serum levels of theophylline are affected by drugs that induce or inhibit hepatic enzymes (see page 12).
- There is a risk of hypokalaemia when theophylline is given with corticosteroids or diuretics.

Inhaled corticosteroids

Mechanism of action

Steroids are potent anti-inflammatory agents, and they reduce bronchial hyperreactivity by:

- Inhibiting the secretion of leukotrienes from lung macrophages
- Reducing the numbers of circulating eosinophils

- Inhibiting the formation of cytokines by lymphocytes and macrophages
- Reducing capillary permeability and oedema
- Inhibiting the accumulation of macrophages at sites of inflammation
- Reducing mucus secretion.

Examples

- Beclometasone
- Budesonide
- Fluticasone.

Example prescriptions

BECLOMETASONE 100 micrograms inhaled b.d.[*]

QVAR 100 ACCUHALER® 1 puff inhaled b.d.[†]

FLIXOTIDE DISKHALER® 250 micrograms inhaled b.d.[‡]

[*]An MDI.
[†]A breath-activated inhaler.
[‡]A dry powder device.

Indication

Prophylaxis of asthma.

Contraindications

None. Care should however be taken not to exceed recommended maximum doses.

Common side effects

- Hoarseness
- Oral candidiasis.

The use of spacer devices and rinsing out the mouth after inhalation of corticosteroids reduce the incidence of these local side effects.

Inhaled corticosteroids have fewer side effects than oral steroids because generally much smaller doses are taken. However, high doses can have significant systemic side effects (see page 184).

Interactions

See page 182.

Mast cell stabilisers

Mechanism of action

Although these agents are called 'mast cell stabilisers', their mode of action is not entirely clear. They do inhibit immediate type 1 hypersensitivity reactions to allergens and also inhibit late-phase reactions. Nedocromil prevents the activation and release of inflammatory mediators, including histamine and leukotriene C_4 (LTC_4) from mast cells and macrophages. These drugs are generally less effective prophylactic agents than inhaled corticosteroids. They can be taken orally or administered by aerosol, nebuliser or dry powder devices.

Examples

- Sodium cromoglicate
- Nedocromil sodium.

Example prescription

SODIUM CROMOGLICATE 20 mg nebulised q.i.d.

Indications

- Prophylaxis of asthma
- Allergic rhinitis
- Allergic conjunctivitis.

Contraindications

None.

Common side effects

- Coughing
- Transient bronchospasm.

Significant interactions

None.

Leukotriene receptor antagonists

The leukotriene receptor antagonists montelukast and zafirlukast are selective high-affinity competive antagonists of the cysteinyl-leukotriene 1 receptor. The cysteinyl leukotrienes are all potent constrictors of bronchial smooth muscle.

Examples
- Montelukast
- Zafirlukast.

Example prescription
> MONTELUKAST 10 mg p.o. o.d

Indication
Prophylaxis of asthma.

Contraindications
- Pregnancy and breast-feeding
- Churg–Strauss syndrome
- Renal impairment
- Hepatic impairment.

Side effects
- Gastrointestinal disturbances
- Hypersensitivity reactions (urticaria and/or angioedema)
- Hepatitis.

Significant interactions
- Plasma concentration of zafirlukast is increased by aspirin.
- Zafirlukast increases the anticoagulant effect of warfarin, and increases the plasma concentration of theophylline.

Oxygen and oxygen delivery systems

Oxygen therapy is the administration of oxygen at concentrations greater than the concentration in ambient air (21%), with the intention of treating or preventing the symptoms and manifestations of hypoxia (inadequate tissue oxygenation). Oxygen is a drug and must be prescribed. Although breathlessness and hypoxaemia may coexist, they are caused by different mechanisms and require different management.

Oxygenation can be assessed in the following ways:

- Clinically: by detection of cyanosis in skin, nail beds and mucosae
- Non-invasively: by pulse oximetry (this indicates the percentage of haemoglobin saturated with oxygen – the Sp_{O_2})
- Invasively: by analysing an arterial blood sample.

Respiratory failure can be diagnosed only on arterial blood gases (ABGs) because there is no non-invasive method for measuring Pa_{CO_2}.

Oxygen delivery devices

The amount of oxygen that a patient actually receives depends on:

- The depth and rate of breathing
- The delivery apparatus used
- The oxygen flow rate.

Fixed performance devices

Fixed performance devices deliver an accurate percentage of oxygen to the patient. Venturi facemasks (Figure 4.2) are commonly used in practice.

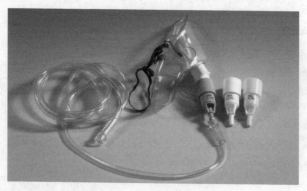

Figure 4.2
Venturi facemask.

The Venturi adapter has a plastic body, with a small jet hole that is attached to the oxygen outlet. The body of the Venturi cone contains holes of varying sizes that allow the entry of room air, which dilutes the oxygen to a fixed concentration. The flow rate required to deliver a fixed concentration of oxygen is written on the cone. Holes in the facemask allow CO_2 to escape. Venturi masks are colour coded and deliver oxygen as shown in Table 4.1.

Venturi mask colour	Inspired oxygen concentration (Fio_2) (%)
Blue	24
White	28
Yellow	35
Red	40
Green	60

Table 4.1 Colour coding of Venturi facemasks

Variable performance devices

Variable performance devices deliver an approximate percentage of oxygen, and should not be used in patients who need an accurate prescription of oxygen, such as patients with type 2 respiratory failure. Variable performance devices in common use include nasal cannulae, intersurgical facemasks and non-rebreathable facemasks.

Nasal cannulae (Figure 4.3) allow the patient to eat and drink and speak more comfortably than they would with a mask. Oxygen flow rates of 1–4 l/minute are used with nasal cannulae. The actual Fio_2 varies with the rate and depth of inhalation, but for most purposes Table 4.2 gives approximate values for the Fio_2. Flow rates higher than 3 l/minute are uncomfortable and cause drying of the nasal mucosa.

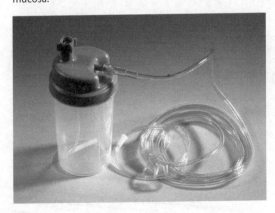

Figure 4.3 Nasal cannulae.

Oxygen flow rate through nasal cannulae (l/min)	Approximate Fio$_2$ (5)
1	24
2	28
3	32

Table 4.2 Approximate levels of inspired oxygen concentration (Fio$_2$)

Intersurgical facemasks (Figure 4.4) are used when higher percentages of oxygen are needed. The actual Fio$_2$ achieved depends on the breathing pattern of the patient; 5–8 l/minute is the range of use. Lower flow rates should not be used because they cause CO_2 retention. For most purposes Table 4.3 gives approximate levels for the Fio$_2$.

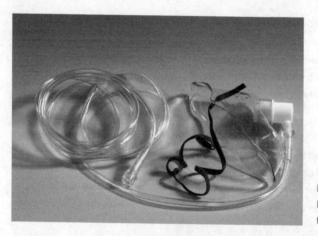

Figure 4.4
Intersurgical
facemask.

Oxygen flow rate through intersurgical facemask (l/min)	Approximate FiO$_2$ (%)
5	35
6	40
8	50

Table 4.3 Approximate levels of the Fio$_2$ for intersurgical facemasks

The non-rebreathable mask (Figure 4.5) delivers high oxygen concentrations through the addition of a reservoir bag and a one-way valve. The flow rate should be kept high enough (8–12 l/minute) to keep the bag inflated; 12 l/minute delivers 99% oxygen.

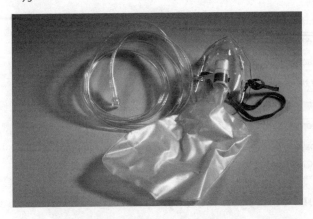

Figure 4.5 Non-rebreathable mask.

Oxygen delivered through Venturi and intersurgical facemasks should *not* be humidified, because moisture condensing in the mask can upset the proportions of the air:oxygen mixture.

Humidification (Figure 4.6) is used in most other delivery systems.

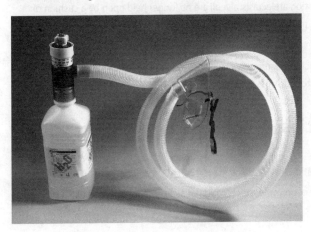

Figure 4.6 Humidified oxygen delivery system.

Long-term oxygen therapy (LTOT; at least 15 hours daily) prolongs survival in some patients with COPD. It is prescribed only after assessment by a respiratory specialist, and is provided via an oxygen concentrator rather than oxygen cylinders.

Indications for oxygen therapy

- Acute emergency situations where hypoxaemia is suspected
- Hypoxaemia (Pao_2 < 8 kPa or Spo_2 < 90%)
- Severe trauma
- Acute myocardial infarction
- Palliation of terminal phase of respiratory tract malignancy
- LTOT: oxygen delivered for 16 hours/day to prevent the symptoms of chronic hypoxia.

Complications of oxygen therapy

- CO_2 narcosis: severe respiratory depression can occur when high concentrations are administered to patients with ventilatory failure who depend on the hypoxic drive to breathe.
- Bronchopulmonary dysplasia and retrolental fibroplasia in pre-term neonates.
- Absorption atelectasis: alveoli are no longer held open by a cushion of inert nitrogen.
- Oxygen is a fire hazard.
- O_2 toxicity: inflammatory response in lungs, which can lead to adult respiratory distress syndrome.

Emergencies

Acute exacerbation of asthma

The management of an acute exacerbation of asthma is summarised in Figure 4.7.

Figure 4.7 Management of acute severe asthma in adults in hospital

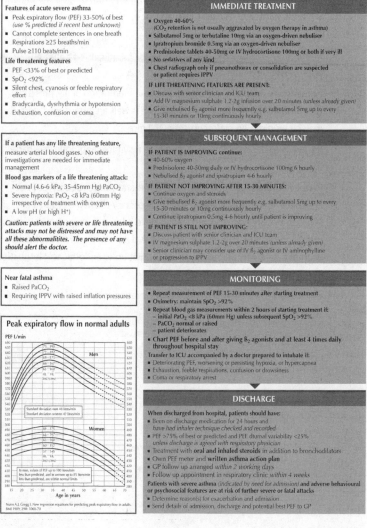

Features of acute severe asthma
- Peak expiratory flow (PEF) 33-50% of best (*use % predicted if recent best unknown*)
- Cannot complete sentences in one breath
- Respirations ≥25 breaths/min
- Pulse ≥110 beats/min

Life threatening features
- PEF <33% of best or predicted
- SpO_2 <92%
- Silent chest, cyanosis or feeble respiratory effort
- Bradycardia, dysrhythmia or hypotension
- Exhaustion, confusion or coma

If a patient has any life threatening feature, measure arterial blood gases. No other investigations are needed for immediate management

Blood gas markers of a life threatening attack:
- Normal (4.6-6 kPa, 35-45mm Hg) $PaCO_2$
- Severe hypoxia: PaO_2 <8 kPa (60mm Hg) irrespective of treatment with oxygen
- A low pH (or high H^+)

Caution: patients with severe or life threatening attacks may not be distressed and may not have all these abnormalities. The presence of any should alert the doctor.

Near fatal asthma
- Raised $PaCO_2$
- Requiring IPPV with raised inflation pressures

Peak expiratory flow in normal adults

Nunn A.J, Gregg I. New regression equations for predicting peak expiratory flow in adults. BMJ 1989; 298: 1068-70

IMMEDIATE TREATMENT
- Oxygen 40-60% (CO_2 retention is not usually aggravated by oxygen therapy in asthma)
- Salbutamol 5mg or terbutaline 10mg via an oxygen-driven nebuliser
- Ipratropium bromide 0.5mg via an oxygen-driven nebuliser
- Prednisolone tablets 40-50mg or IV hydrocortisone 100mg or both if very ill
- No sedatives of any kind
- Chest radiograph only if pneumothorax or consolidation are suspected or patient requires IPPV

IF LIFE THREATENING FEATURES ARE PRESENT:
- Discuss with senior clinician and ICU team
- Add IV magnesium sulphate 1.2-2g infusion over 20 minutes (*unless already given*)
- Give nebulised β₂ agonist more frequently e.g. salbutamol 5mg up to every 15-30 minutes or 10mg continuously hourly

SUBSEQUENT MANAGEMENT

IF PATIENT IS IMPROVING continue:
- 40-60% oxygen
- Prednisolone 40-50mg daily or IV hydrocortisone 100mg 6 hourly
- Nebulised β₂ agonist and ipratropium 4-6 hourly

IF PATIENT NOT IMPROVING AFTER 15-30 MINUTES:
- Continue oxygen and steroids
- Give nebulised β₂ agonist more frequently e.g. salbutamol 5mg up to every 15-30 minutes or 10mg continuously hourly
- Continue ipratropium 0.5mg 4-6 hourly until patient is improving

IF PATIENT IS STILL NOT IMPROVING:
- Discuss patient with senior clinician and ICU team
- IV magnesium sulphate 1.2-2g over 20 minutes (*unless already given*)
- Senior clinician may consider use of IV β₂ agonist or IV aminophylline or progression to IPPV

MONITORING
- Repeat measurement of PEF 15-30 minutes after starting treatment
- Oximetry: maintain SpO_2 >92%
- Repeat blood gas measurements within 2 hours of starting treatment if:
  – initial PaO_2 <8 kPa (60mm Hg) unless subsequent SpO_2 >92%,
  – $PaCO_2$ normal or raised
  – patient deteriorates
- Chart PEF before and after giving β₂ agonists and at least 4 times daily throughout hospital stay

Transfer to ICU accompanied by a doctor prepared to intubate if:
- Deteriorating PEF, worsening or persisting hypoxia, or hypercapnea
- Exhaustion, feeble respirations, confusion or drowsiness
- Coma or respiratory arrest

DISCHARGE

When discharged from hospital, patients should have:
- Been on discharge medication for 24 hours and *have had inhaler technique checked and recorded*
- PEF >75% of best or predicted and PEF diurnal variability <25% *unless discharge is agreed with respiratory physician*
- Treatment with **oral and inhaled steroids** in addition to bronchodilators
- Own PEF meter and **written asthma action plan**
- GP follow up arranged *within 2 working days*
- Follow up appointment in respiratory clinic *within 4 weeks*

Patients with severe asthma (*indicated by need for admission*) **and adverse behavioural or psychosocial features are at risk of further severe or fatal attacks**
- Determine reason(s) for exacerbation and admission
- Send details of admission, discharge and potential best PEF to GP

Reproduced with the kind permission of the Scottish Intercollegiate Guidelines Network and British Thoracic Society. Taken from the British Thoracic Society *Thorax*, 2003; **58** (Suppl 1): i1-i92.

Acute infective exacerbation of COPD

- Administer controlled oxygen therapy using a Venturi mask. If the patient is known to have COPD, start with an Fio_2 of 28%.

- Give nebulised bronchodilators, eg salbutamol 5 mg and ipratropium bromide 500 micrograms. These may require a repeat dose after an appropriate time interval.

- Administer a steroid. If the patient can take medication orally, prescribe prednisolone, eg 40 mg. If the patient is less well, an intravenous steroid may be required, eg hydrocortisone 200 mg.

- If there is evidence of infection, prescribe a suitable antibiotic (see page 265).

- Perform ABG analysis and titrate oxygen therapy as required. Frequent checks of ABG concentrations may be necessary to enable optimal gas levels to be achieved. The aim is to achieve adequate oxygenation without unacceptable hypercapnia and acidosis. A deterioration in ABGs should prompt assessment for non-invasive ventilation or endotracheal intubation and mechanical ventilation.

- Physiotherapy can be used to aid expectoration, which can improve respiratory function.

5
Alimentary system

Antacids
Ulcer-healing drugs
H. pylori eradication
Anti-emetics
Anti-inflammatory drugs for inflammatory bowel disease
Anti-motility drugs
Anti-spasmodics
Drugs affecting bile
Laxatives
Pancreatin
Management of upper gastrointestinal tract haemorrhage
Management of ascites

5
Alimentary system

Antacids

Essential physiology

In health, the oesophageal mucosa is protected from the damaging effects of acidic gastric contents by a variety of physical mechanisms that prevent the gastric contents from refluxing upwards. The lower oesophageal sphincter plays a major role in this process (Figure 5.1).

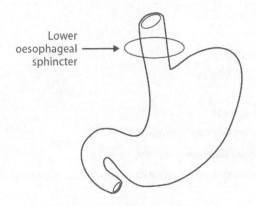

Lower oesophageal sphincter →

Figure 5.1 Basic anatomy, showing the lower oesophageal sphincter.

In gastro-oesophageal reflux disease (GORD), anti-reflux mechanisms are defective. Irritating gastric contents can therefore come into contact with the oesophageal mucosa, which may result in oesophagitis and, in the long term, a premalignant condition called Barrett's oesophagus.

The two antacids most commonly used are aluminium salts and magnesium salts.

Aluminium and magnesium salts

Mechanism of action

These compounds are weak bases that neutralise gastric acid, thereby raising the pH in the stomach. The enzyme pepsin (which can irritate the stomach and oesophagus) works best in acidic conditions. Antacids therefore indirectly reduce its activity.

Examples

- Aluminium hydroxide
- Magnesium carbonate.

Example prescription

ALUMINIUM HYDROXIDE 500 mg chewed q.i.d.

Indications

- Dyspepsia
- GORD.

Contraindications

Hypophosphataemia.

Common side effects

- Aluminium salts cause constipation.
- Magnesium salts cause diarrhoea.

Combined aluminium/magnesium preparations may help counteract each other's side effects.

Significant interactions

- Antacids can impair the absorption of many other drugs, especially tetracyclines and iron.
- They make urine more alkaline, with the result that acidic drugs (such as aspirin) can be excreted in increased amounts.
- Antacids can damage the enteric coating on other medications.

Compound alginates

Alginic acid-containing antacids raise the gastric pH in a similar manner to regular antacids (Figure 5.2). In addition, alginate forms a 'raft' that floats on top of the gastric contents and acts as a physical barrier to prevent reflux into the oesophagus.

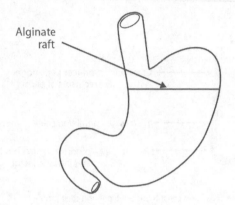

Figure 5.2 Mechanism of action of compound alginates.

Ulcer-healing drugs

Essential physiology

The stomach is composed of a variety of cell types, each with its own specialised function. Figure 5.3 shows a typical gastric pit in the fundus of the stomach. Note the four main cell types and their products.

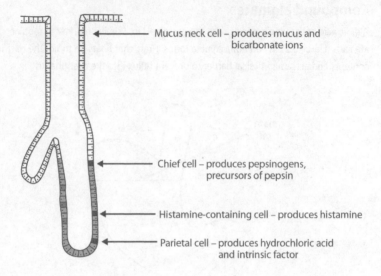

Figure 5.3 A gastric pit, indicating constituent cell types and their products.

A further specialised cell type – the G-cell – is found in the antrum and produces gastrin.

The inner workings of the parietal cell are particularly relevant. In the resting state (ie when not secreting acid), parietal cells contain tubulovesicular structures with H^+/K^+ ATPase (adenosine triphosphatase) pumps in their walls. Activation of these structures can occur by several mechanisms, but all result in the same outcome – movement of the pump to the apical membrane of the cell with the subsequent pumping of H^+ into the gastric lumen. Chloride ions are also transferred (by a different mechanism) and the two ions combine to form hydrochloric acid. The control mechanisms for this process are shown in Figure 5.4.

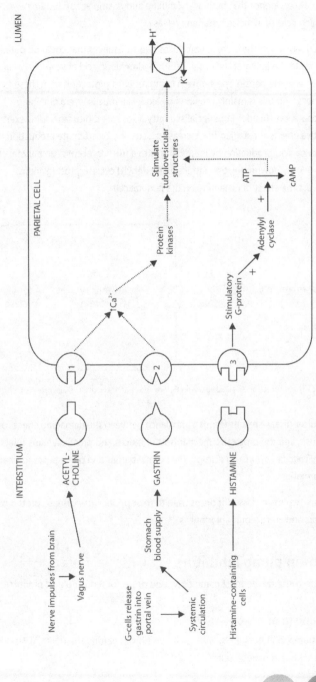

Figure 5.4 Control mechanisms for acid secretion from parietal cells: (1) acetylcholine muscarinic (M_3) receptor; (2) gastrin receptor; (3) histamine (H_2) receptor; and (4) H^+/K^+ ATPase pump.

There is also evidence that both acetylcholine and gastrin act on histamine-containing cells to increase histamine release.

As described above, the stomach produces two substances that could be potentially damaging to the lining of the organ itself – hydrochloric acid at very low pH and the digestive enzyme pepsin. The stomach lining requires protection from these substances, and this is mainly provided by a gel-like mucus layer containing bicarbonate ions. In addition, specialised fatty acids called prostaglandins exert protective effects. Prostaglandins increase mucus and bicarbonate production, and also reduce acid production by interacting with a further receptor on parietal cells (Figure 5.5). By downregulating intracellular adenylyl cyclase, prostaglandins counteract the effect of histamine on the parietal cell.

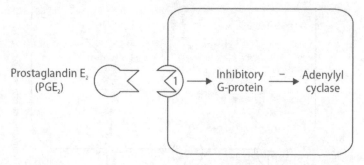

Figure 5.5 The interaction of prostaglandin E_2 with the parietal cell: (1) PGE_2 receptor.

Peptic ulcer disease results from an imbalance between the damaging effects of acid and pepsin and the protective mechanisms of mucus and prostaglandins. Infection with *Helicobacter pylori* also disrupts the normal barrier and predisposes to peptic ulcer formation.

There are two main classes of drugs used to treat peptic ulcer disease, proton pump inhibitors and H_2-receptor antagonists.

1. Proton pump inhibitors

These are currently the most commonly used drugs for reducing acid production.

Mechanism of action

Proton pump inhibitors (PPIs) work by irreversibly inhibiting the H^+/K^+ ATPase pump (proton pump) in parietal cells.

Examples

- Omeprazole
- Lansoprazole
- Pantoprazole.

Example prescription

LANSOPRAZOLE 30 mg p.o. o.d.

Indications

- Peptic ulcer disease
- GORD
- Dyspepsia
- *H. pylori* eradication (see below)
- Zollinger–Ellison syndrome
- Reducing acid secretion during general anaesthesia.

Absolute contraindications

None.

Relative contraindications

These drugs should be used with caution in liver disease, pregnancy and breast-feeding.

Common side effects

- Gastrointestinal disturbances, especially diarrhoea
- Headache
- Dizziness.

Significant interactions

Omeprazole is an inhibitor of the cytochrome P450 enzyme system and thus may have many interactions (see page 12).

2. H$_2$-receptor antagonists

Mechanism of action

These drugs are competitive inhibitors of histamine-induced acid secretion.

Examples

- Ranitidine
- Cimetidine.

Example prescription

RANITIDINE 150 mg p.o. b.d.

Indications

- Peptic ulcer disease
- GORD
- Dyspepsia
- *H. pylori* eradication (see below)
- Zollinger–Ellison syndrome
- Reducing acid secretion during general anaesthesia.

Absolute contraindications

None.

Relative contraindications

These drugs should be used with caution in kidney disease, liver disease, pregnancy and breast-feeding.

Common side effects

- Gastrointestinal disturbances, especially diarrhoea
- Headache
- Dizziness
- Derangement of liver function tests.

Significant interactions

Cimetidine is an inhibitor of the cytochrome P450 enzyme system, and thus may have many interactions (see page 12).

Other drugs

Misoprostol

This is a synthetic prostaglandin analogue, which may be used to mimic the activity of endogenous prostaglandins, thus improving the stomach's resistance to damage. This agent is most often co-prescribed with a non-steroidal anti-inflammatory drug (NSAID) such as diclofenac, to reduce NSAID-induced ulceration.

Tripotassium dicitratobismuthate

This is a bismuth chelate that adheres to the base of an ulcer and promotes ulcer healing.

Sucralfate

This is a complex of aluminium and sucrose, which also binds to the base of an ulcer and promotes healing.

H. pylori eradication

Infection of the stomach with the Gram-negative bacillus *H. pylori* predisposes to the development of peptic ulcer disease. Testing for the presence of the organism should be carried out in all patients with a peptic ulcer, and eradication should be attempted in affected individuals. There is some evidence that eradication therapy should be given to all patients with a peptic ulcer, regardless of their *H. pylori* status.

There is a wide variety of treatment regimens aimed at eradicating infection, which combine an ulcer-healing drug with antibacterial agents. The two most commonly used regimens are as follows:

- Lansoprazole 30 mg b.d., clarithromycin 500 mg b.d. and amoxicillin 1 g b.d. for 7–14 days
- Lansoprazole 30 mg b.d., clarithromycin 500 mg b.d. and metronidazole 500 mg b.d. for 7 days.

The second combination is often used if the first is ineffective in clearing the infection.

Antiemetics

Essential physiology

The act of vomiting (emesis) is a complex process that is coordinated by the vomiting centre in the medulla oblongata. Vomiting is usually associated with nausea. During an act of vomiting, the vomiting centre coordinates respiration, gastrointestinal motility and abdominal wall muscle contraction to propel gastric contents towards the mouth, while attempting to keep the airway patent.

The vomiting centre has four main inputs, which can act alone or in combination to result in vomiting (Figure 5.6).

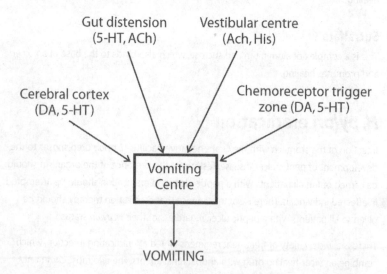

Figure 5.6 Main inputs into the vomiting centre. ACh, acetylcholine; DA, dopamine; His, histamine; 5-hydroxytryptamine 5-HT (serotonin).

Gastrointestinal tract irritation or distension

Ingestion of irritating substances (eg alcohol) and distension of the gastrointestinal tract (eg gastric distension with pyloric stenosis) cause activation of the vomiting centre. Serotonin (5-hydroxytryptophan or 5-HT) and acetylcholine are important mediators of this process.

Vestibular centre

The vestibular apparatus in the inner ear is responsible for the nausea and vomiting that can accompany motion (motion sickness). Acetylcholine and histamine are important mediators.

Cerebral cortex

Inputs to the vomiting centre from the diencephalon and limbic system account for the fact that emotional upset and pain can result in vomiting. Dopamine and 5-HT are important mediators.

Chemoreceptor trigger zone

This is a specialised area of brain found near the fourth ventricle. Metabolic upsets (eg uraemia) and nauseating drugs are detected here. Dopamine and 5-HT are important mediators.

Drugs that can cause nausea and vomiting include:

- Chemotherapy drugs
- Dopamine agonists, eg L-dopa
- Opioid analgesics
- Digoxin
- Selective serotonin reuptake inhibitors (SSRIs).

There are four classes of antiemetics commonly in use: antihistamines, prokinetic agents, serotonin 5-HT, receptor antagonists and dopamine D_2 receptor antagonists.

Antihistamines

Mechanism of action

These drugs block the action of histamine on H_1 receptors and are thus particularly effective in treating nausea and vomiting caused by vestibular disturbances. They can also be effective in treating nausea and vomiting resulting from other causes. In addition to their effects on histamine receptors, most of these agents are antagonists at muscarinic acetylcholine receptors.

Example

Cyclizine.

Example prescription

CYCLIZINE 50 mg p.o. t.i.d.

Common side effects

- Drowsiness
- Anti-muscarinic effects, eg urinary retention, dry mouth, blurred vision.

Prokinetic agents

Mechanism of action

These agents act to promote gastrointestinal motility and speed transit through the gut. They are therefore particularly helpful in cases of gut distension. In addition to this effect, metoclopramide and domperidone act as dopamine receptor antagonists and metoclopramide is an antagonist at serotonin 5-HT$_3$ receptors.

Examples

- Metoclopramide
- Domperidone.

Example prescription

METOCLOPRAMIDE 10 mg p.o. 8-hourly p.r.n. Max. 30 mg per day

Contraindications

Gastrointestinal obstruction, perforation, haemorrhage.

Common side effects

- Extrapyramidal effects (parkinsonism, akathisia, dystonias and tardive dyskinesia)
- Hyperprolactinaemia.

Serotonin 5-HT₃ receptor antagonists

Mechanism of action

By blocking the 5-HT_3 serotonin receptor, these agents block many of the inputs into the vomiting centre. They are highly effective antiemetics and are particularly useful in treating nausea and vomiting caused by chemotherapy.

Example

Ondansetron.

Example prescription

ONDANSETRON 4 mg p.o. 8-hourly p.r.n.

Common side effects

· Constipation
· Flushing.

Dopamine D₂ receptor antagonists

Mechanism of action

This class includes phenothiazine anti-psychotic drugs, which are described on page 135. The antiemetic property is a result of antagonism of dopamine receptors in the chemoreceptor trigger zone. As a result of their side-effect profile, these agents should not be used routinely as antiemetics.

Other drugs

· Corticosteroids are often used in combination with serotonin 5-HT_3 receptor antagonists in patients receiving chemotherapy.
· Cannabinoids (eg nabilone) have antiemetic effects.
· Anxiolytic agents (eg benzodiazepines) may also act as antiemetics, although this property may simply be a result of their relaxing effects.

Anti-inflammatory drugs for inflammatory bowel disease

Essential physiology

Complex pathophysiological pathways govern the inflammation in inflammatory bowel disease (IBD). The exact mechanism of action of many of the anti-inflammatory drugs used in the treatment of such conditions is not known (see page 182 for the mechanisms underpinning corticosteroid usage).

Aminosalicylates

There are a variety of these drugs in common use. They are generally used in an attempt to maintain remission from active IBD.

Mechanism of action

These compounds work by delivering 5-aminosalicylic acid (5-ASA) to the bowel. The exact mechanism of action of this agent is not fully understood; however, scavenging of free radicals may play a significant role. The members of this class of drug differ in the way in which 5-ASA is delivered to the bowel.

Examples

- Sulfasalazine: a combination of 5-ASA and sulfapyridine
- Mesalazine: 5-ASA only
- Balsalazide: 5-ASA in a pro-drug formulation
- Olsalazine: a 5-ASA dimer.

Example prescription

BALSALAZIDE 2.25 g p.o. t.i.d.

Indication

Mild-to-moderate IBD (generally used for ulcerative colitis, but sulfasalazine can also be used in Crohn's disease).

Common side effects

- Gastrointestinal upset
- Hypersensitivity reactions
- Blood disorders (eg agranulocytosis, aplastic anaemia and thrombocytopenia).

Patients should be advised to attend a doctor should they experience any symptoms of a blood dyscrasia (eg easy bruising, unexplained bleeding or fever).

Other drugs

Corticosteroids

The mechanism of action of these agents is described on page 182. Steroids can be given orally or as rectal preparations in the treatment of IBD. They are particularly useful in relapses of IBD.

Cytokine inhibitors

Infliximab is a monoclonal antibody that is active against tumour necrosis factor (TNF-α). It is becoming increasingly important in the management of severe IBD. The drug is given by intravenous infusion once every 4–6 weeks to induce remission. See page 216.

Other agents

Azathioprine and 6-mercaptopurine can be used in an attempt to minimise glucocorticosteroid use (see page 241). Ciclosporin and methotrexate are also used infrequently.

Anti-motility drugs

The mainstay of treatment for diarrhoea is rehydration. Occasionally, antibiotics are required when diarrhoea is caused by a bacterial infection. Antimotility drugs should be used sparingly and are generally not recommended for acute diarrhoeal states.

Mechanism of action

The antimotility agents in common use are opiates or derivatives of opiates. Their receptor target is the μ opiate receptor, although they may have actions on serotonin and acetylcholine pathways. They act to reduce gut peristalsis and may also increase absorption.

Examples

- Codeine phosphate
- Loperamide hydrochloride.

Example prescription

LOPERAMIDE 4 mg p.o. b.d.

Contraindications

- Acute colitis
- Abdominal distension.

Common side effects

- Abdominal cramps
- Nausea and vomiting.

Anti-spasmodics

Essential physiology

The autonomic nervous system (ANS) plays an important role in the control of normal motility in the gastrointestinal tract. In a 'fight or flight' situation, the sympathetic nervous system (SNS) is activated. This acts to slow down transit through the gut. In contrast, parasympathetic activity results in activation of the gut, with contraction of the gut wall and relaxation of sphincters.

The parasympathetic nervous system (PNS) relies on acetylcholine as a neurotransmitter. This substance acts on muscarinic acetylcholine receptors in target organs to generate a response.

Mechanism of action

Most antispasmodics are 'anti-muscarinic' compounds, in that they act to block the effect of acetylcholine on muscarinic receptors. In so doing, these agents attenuate the effect of the PNS on the gut, thereby reducing its motility.

Examples

- Hyoscine butylbromide
- Dicycloverine hydrochloride.

Example prescription

HYOSCINE BUTYLBROMIDE 20 mg p.o. q.i.d.

Indication

Relief from gastrointestinal spasm (ie cramps).

Contraindications

- Any condition hindering gastrointestinal transit, eg paralytic ileus
- Angle-closure glaucoma
- Myasthenia gravis
- Enlarged prostate gland.

Common side effects

All side effects are predictable, bearing in mind that the mechanism of action involves blocking of the PNS:

- Tachycardia
- Constipation
- Urinary retention
- Dry mouth.

Other drugs

A number of other agents are used as antispasmodics. These include alverine citrate and mebeverine hydrochloride, which both relax smooth muscle in the bowel wall.

Drugs affecting bile

Essential physiology

Bile is synthesised by liver hepatocytes. It may be stored in the gallbladder before being released into the duodenum, where bile salts play an important role in the digestion and absorption of fat. The body recycles bile salts to reduce the amount of synthesis necessary. The recycling process is known as 'enterohepatic recirculation', and involves reabsorption of bile salts from the distal ileum.

Pruritis is often a troublesome symptom in patients with jaundice. It is caused by the deposition of bile salts in the skin. Defective reabsorption of bile salts, as can occur in Crohn's disease, can contribute to diarrhoea.

Colestyramine

Mechanism of action

This is an anion exchange resin that binds bile salts in the intestine. It can therefore reduce itch in jaundice (as fewer bile salts are reabsorbed) and reduce diarrhoea in various conditions (eg Crohn's disease and post-ileal resection).

Example prescription

COLESTYRAMINE 4 g p.o o.d.

Indications

- Pruritus caused by biliary obstruction and primary biliary cirrhosis
- Selected cases of diarrhoea.

Common side effects

Constipation.

Significant interactions

- The absorption of many drugs can be affected, so this drug should not be administered at the same time as other medications.

Laxatives

Essential physiology

Normal bowel motility depends on the complex interaction between various hormone and nervous system inputs. The precise mechanisms are poorly understood. Disruption of normal bowel contractions can result in constipation.

There are four main classes of laxatives (bulk-forming, osmotic, stimulant and faecal softeners). Some drugs have properties from more than one class.

Bulk-forming laxatives

Mechanism of action

These drugs absorb water, and increase the volume of faeces in the colon. They thereby stimulate peristalsis. They are given orally.

Examples

- Bran
- Ispaghula husk
- Methylcellulose
- Sterculia.

Example prescription

FYBOGEL® 3.5 g p.o b.d.

Osmotic laxatives

Mechanism of action

These agents are poorly absorbed and draw fluid into the bowel by osmosis. They therefore increase the volume of faeces and stimulate peristalsis. In addition, magnesium salts increase the secretion of cholecystokinin, which increases motility and fluid secretion. Most are administered orally.

Examples

- Lactulose
- Macrogols
- Magnesium hydroxide
- Phosphates (given rectally)
- Sodium citrate (given rectally).

Example prescription

LACTULOSE 15 ml p.o. b.d.

Stimulant laxatives

Mechanism of action

This is incompletely understood. These agents may damage the gut wall and can interfere with hormone systems, thus altering bowel motility. They should not be used long term. Glycerol suppositories work by directly irritating the rectal wall.

Examples

- Bisacodyl (given orally or rectally)
- Senna (an anthraquinone laxative) (given orally)
- Sodium picosulfate (given orally)
- Glycerol (given rectally).

Example prescription

GLYCEROL 1 suppository p.r. stat

Faecal softeners

Mechanism of action

These act to soften hard stools, to ease their passage.

Examples

- Docusate sodium (this also has stimulant laxative properties) (given orally or rectally)
- Arachis oil (given rectally)
- Liquid paraffin (given orally).

Example prescription

ARACHIS OIL 130 ml p.r. stat

Shared properties of laxatives

Indication

Constipation.

Contraindications

- Dysphagia
- Intestinal obstruction
- Atonic colon
- Faecal impaction
- Arachis oil is contraindicated in patients with allergy to peanuts.

Common side effects

- Flatulence
- Abdominal distension and cramps
- Gastrointestinal obstruction
- Faecal impaction
- Liquid paraffin: causes anal irritation
- Melanosis coli: a blackened appearance of the bowel mucosa resulting from chronic use of senna and other anthraquinone laxatives.

Significant interactions

None.

Pancreatin

Essential physiology

Normally, when food enters the small intestine, hormones (secretin and cholecystokinin) are released that trigger the release of pancreatic enzymes. Pancreatic enzymes include various proteases, peptidases, lipase and amylase, which degrade ingested food.

Exocrine pancreatic deficiency occurs in a number of disease states, eg:

- Cystic fibrosis
- Chronic pancreatitis
- After a pancreatectomy.

In such cases, malabsorption will occur unless pancreatic enzymes are given as supplements.

Mechanism of action

Pancreatin preparations contain varying amounts of exocrine pancreatic enzymes. They aim to replace deficient enzymes in the small bowel. As the enzymes are inactivated at low pH, these supplements are best taken with food or after the administration of an agent to raise gastric pH.

Example prescription

CREON® 25 000 – 1 capsule p.o. with meals

Common side effects

- Oral irritation
- Nausea and vomiting
- Abdominal discomfort.

Management of upper gastrointestinal tract haemorrhage

Upper gastrointestinal tract haemorrhage is traditionally divided into variceal (or presumed variceal) and non-variceal haemorrhage.

Initial management of the two subtypes is identical, and incorporates the emergency measures that one would adopt when faced with any acutely unwell patient.

Non-variceal bleeding

The 'ABC' approach is used: first the **a**irway is assessed and secured, and high-flow oxygen applied. A rapid assessment of **b**reathing follows. Management of the **c**irculation will obviously require most attention. Patients will range from being haemodynamically stable to being in severe shock, and management should be tailored to suit the patient.

Intravenous access must be obtained, ideally with two large-bore venous cannulae. Blood samples can often be taken at the time of cannulation. At the very least, blood should be sent for: full blood count, coagulation profile, renal function and electrolyte profile, liver function, glucose, and group and cross-match. Fluid resuscitation must begin without delay. Catastrophic bleeds will require resuscitation with packed red cells. Ideally, blood should be cross-matched. Type-specific blood (ie matched to the patient's blood group, but not actually cross-matched) would be a second best option. In emergency situations, however, there may not be time for laboratory analysis, and group O rhesus-negative blood can be used as an interim measure. Other blood products may be required to correct coagulopathies or low platelet levels.

Monitor the patient's response to fluid resuscitation with frequent observations of respiratory rate, pulse rate, blood pressure, perfusion of the peripheries, conscious level and urine output. More invasive monitoring may be required, and this is usually performed in a high dependency or intensive care setting.

Consideration should be given to performing upper gastrointestinal endoscopy at the earliest possible opportunity to identify the cause of the bleeding and to allow more directed therapy.

Variceal bleeding

Bleeding from varices carries a higher mortality rate than non-variceal bleeding. Initial resuscitation in a patient with suspected varices should be as documented above.

If upper gastrointestinal endoscopy is available, this should be performed as soon as possible. Variceal bleeding may be controlled by banding or injecting (sclerotherapy) the varices. In cases where bleeding cannot be controlled by these measures, balloon tamponade, a transjugular intrahepatic portosystemic shunt (TIPS) or surgery may be considered.

If upper gastrointestinal endoscopy is not readily available, medical management of variceal bleeding is adopted. Two main options are available: (1) vasopressin or terlipressin ± nitroglycerin and (2) somatostatin and octreotide.

Vasopressin or terlipressin ± nitroglycerin

Vasopressin (antidiuretic hormone or ADH) acts on the collecting ducts in the kidney, resulting in an increase in water permeability. This, in turn, allows water to be reabsorbed and less to be lost in the urine. It also acts to contract smooth muscle. This agent reduces portal blood flow and variceal pressure, and can therefore help to control variceal bleeding. Terlipressin is a vasopressin analogue that has similar actions. Either of these agents can be combined with nitroglycerin. Administration of glypressin in patients with variceal bleeding has been associated with reduced mortality.

Example prescription

TERLIPRESSIN 2 mg i.v. stat followed by 1–2 mg 4–6 hourly until bleeding is controlled, for up to 72 hours.

Somatostatin and octreotide

Somatostatin is a naturally occurring hormone found in the pancreas and central nervous system. Octreotide is a synthetic form with a longer duration of action. These agents can reduce portal pressure and blood flow, and may help to control variceal bleeding.

All patients with variceal bleeding should receive antibiotic prophylaxis, generally with ciprofloxacin (unless there is a contraindication). This can reduce the incidence of spontaneous bacterial peritonitis in these patients.

Ref: BSG Guidelines, 2000, www.bsg.org.uk

Management of ascites

Paracentesis should be performed in all patients with newly detected ascites, unless there is a significant associated coagulopathy. Analysis of ascitic fluid provides important information about the cause of the ascites and can detect infection.

The vast majority of cases of ascites occur in the setting of liver cirrhosis. The management of ascites in other situations may be different to that described below.

Daily sodium intake should be reduced to a maximum of 88 mmol/day. Diuretics are then used in an attempt to clear the fluid. Furosemide and spironolactone are conventionally given in combination, with starting doses of 40 mg o.d. p.o. and 100 mg o.d. p.o. respectively. The doses can be increased every 3–5 days to achieve adequate fluid clearance. When escalating doses, the ratio of the dose of furosemide to that of spironolactone should be kept at 4:10. Usual maximum doses are 160 mg furosemide and 400 mg spironolactone. Diuretics should be stopped if encephalopathy, significant hyponatraemia or renal impairment occur.

Tense ascites should be relieved using a single large-volume paracentesis before resorting to the above medical measures. Refractory ascites is ascites that is unresponsive to diet and diuretics or that recurs rapidly after paracentesis. In such circumstances, serial paracentesis, liver transplantation, insertion of a TIPS or the insertion of a peritoneovenous shunt may be considered.

Ref: Hepatology 2004, **39**, 1–16

6
Neurological system

6 Neurological system

Hypnotics and anxiolytics

Most drugs that reduce anxiety (anxiolytics or sedatives) will induce sleep. Similarly, hypnotic drugs designed to aid sleep will often have an anxiolytic effect. Long-term use of such drugs can lead to physical and psychological dependence with consequent difficulty in drug withdrawal. Always remember that insomnia and anxiety are symptoms, not diagnoses, so management requires investigation and treatment of the cause.

> **Don't forget**
>
> **Hypnotics should be used only for the short-term relief of anxiety or insomnia.**

Essential physiology

Gamma-aminobutyric acid (GABA) is an inhibitory neurotransmitter that functions in many areas of the central nervous system (CNS). There are two types of GABA receptors, $GABA_A$ and $GABA_B$. It is important to know about the former. These receptors are closely linked to Cl^- (chloride) channels as shown in Figure 6.1.

Binding of GABA to its receptor increases the permeability of the channel to Cl^-. Increased Cl^- passage results in a cancelling-out effect on excitatory neurotransmitter activity.

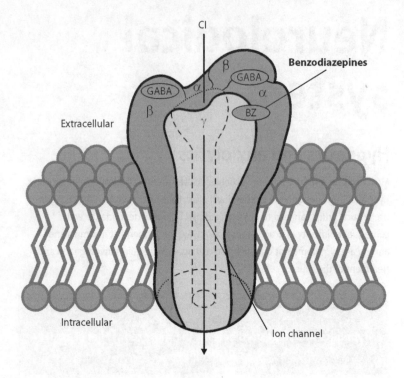

Figure 6.1 A GABA (γ-aminobutyric acid) receptor.

Benzodiazepines

Benzodiazepines are the class of drugs most commonly used as anxiolytics and hypnotics. They are also sometimes used as anticonvulsants. The drugs in this class vary in terms of their half-lives. Benzodiazepines useful as anticonvulsants have a long half-life. A short elimination half-life is desirable for those used as hypnotics.

Mechanism of action

Benzodiazepines bind to specific benzodiazepine receptors that are closely linked to $GABA_A$ receptors and Cl^- channels. They facilitate the action of GABA.

Examples

- Diazepam
- Temazepam
- Chlordiazepoxide
- Lorazepam
- Nitrazepam
- Midazolam.

Example prescriptions

For insomnia:

TEMAZEPAM 10 mg p.o. nocte

For anxiety:

DIAZEPAM 2 mg p.o. t.i.d.

Indications

- Short-term management of insomnia
- Short-term management of anxiety
- Short-term use as a muscle relaxant
- Alcohol withdrawal syndrome (usually chlordiazepoxide)
- Status epilepticus (usually diazepam or lorazepam)
- Panic disorders – acute attacks (usually lorazepam)
- Preoperative sedation and amnesia (usually midazolam or lorazepam).

Absolute contraindications

- Respiratory depression or failure.

Relative contraindications

- Muscle weakness
- Hepatic or renal impairment.

Common side effects

- Impaired judgement and reaction time (patients should be warned not to drive)

- Hangover effect next day: drowsiness and light-headedness
- Confusion: especially in elderly people
- Ataxia
- Respiratory depression in high doses.

Significant interactions

- Increased sedative effect with alcohol, antipsychotics and opioid analgesics
- Enhanced hypotensive effects when given with all classes of antihypertensive drugs.

Other drugs

Zopiclone and zolpidem

These are short-acting non-benzodiazepine hypnotics. Although their molecular structure does not resemble that of the benzodiazepines, these drugs are also thought to have agonist effects on benzodiazepine receptors.

Example prescription

Zoplicone 7.5 mg p.o. nocte

Antipsychotic drugs

Antipsychotic drugs, which are also known as neuroleptics, have a tranquillising effect at doses that do not impair consciousness. They can be given short term for disturbed behaviour in conditions such as mania, delirium, organic brain disease or very severe anxiety. The drugs are used long term for schizophrenia. Newer antipsychotics, the 'atypical' antipsychotics (eg olanzapine), are so-called because they are thought to have fewer side effects than older drugs. Their mechanism of action via actions on dopamine receptors is no different from older anti-psychotic agents, and although they cause less severe effects on the extrapyramidal nervous system, they have more metabolic side effects. Atypical antipsychotics are now used as first-line treatment in newly diagnosed schizophrenia. Antipsychotic drugs can be given orally or parenterally. Long-acting depot intramuscular preparations are sometimes given when there are problems with compliance or intolerance of oral medication.

Essential physiology

In psychotic illness there is disordered thinking and perception. There is no simple aetiological hypothesis. Although it is known that drugs that reduce dopaminergic transmission in the brain reduce some of the features of schizophrenia, such as hallucinations and delusions, it does not follow that the disease is caused by excessive dopamine function.

There are two main classes of drug used for psychotic illnesses, phenothiazines and atypical antipsychotics.

Phenothiazines

Mechanism of action

Virtually all antipsychotic drugs block dopamine D_2 receptors and reduce dopamine neurotransmission in the forebrain. Some agents also interact with dopaminergic D_1 and D_4 receptors, serotoninergic 5-HT_{2A} and 5-HT_{2C} receptors and α-adrenergic receptors. The side effects of these drugs also result from of interaction with these receptors.

Examples

- Chlorpromazine
- Promazine
- Thioridazine
- Prochlorperazine
- Fluphenazine.

Example prescriptions

CHLORPROMAZINE 50 mg p.o. t.i.d.

MODECATE® 50 mg i.m. monthly

Indications

- Acute psychomotor agitation
- Schizophrenia
- Nausea in palliative care
- Hiccups
- Acute vestibular disorders.

Absolute contraindications

CNS depression and coma.

Relative contraindications

- Hepatic impairment
- Cardiac disease, especially long Q–T syndrome
- Parkinson's disease.

Common side effects

- Extrapyramidal effects: parkinsonism, dystonia, akathisia, tardive dyskinesia
- Hypotension
- Neuroleptic malignant syndrome: not common, but serious; comprises hyperthermia, rigidity, fluctuating consciousness level, muscle rigidity and tachycardia
- Galactorrhoea and menstrual disturbances caused by raised serum prolactin
- Photosensitivity, slate-grey skin, skin rash
- Cholestatic jaundice
- ECG changes and arrhythmias.

Interactions

- Enhanced hypotensive effects of antihypertensives
- Ventricular arrhythmias when used with any other drug associated with prolonged Q–T interval, eg anti-arrhythmic drugs, macrolide antibiotics, terfenadine
- Potentiation of the effect of sedatives, analgesics and alcohol.

Atypical antipsychotics

These more recently developed drugs have less risk of extrapyramidal side effects than the phenothiazines. They do carry their own range of adverse effects, however.

Mechanism of action

As for phenothiazines.

Examples

- Risperidone
- Quetiapine
- Olanzapine
- Clozapine: this is used only if there has been no response to the other antipsychotics, because of its risk of blood dyscrasias.

Example prescription

QUETIAPINE 25 mg p.o. b.d.

Indications

- Schizophrenia
- Acute psychosis.

Absolute contraindications

Pregnancy and breast-feeding.

Relative contraindications

- Cardiac disease with arrhythmias
- Epilepsy
- Hepatic or renal impairment.

Common side effects

- Weight gain
- Dizziness and postural hypotension
- Diabetes mellitus (type 2 and ketoacidosis)
- Extrapyramidal, but less than with older psychotropics
- Raised prolactin, but less than with phenothiazines
- Agranulocytosis and cardiomyopathy with clozapine.

Significant interactions

As for phenothiazines.

Other antipsychotics

Haloperidol is a butyrophenone. It is used in patients with psychoses, and for acute agitation and restlessness in elderly people. It is less sedating and has fewer anti-muscarinic and hypotensive side effects than the phenothiazines, but dystonic side effects are more common.

Antidepressants

These drugs are used in depression that is unresponsive to psychological therapy.

Essential physiology

Most antidepressants affect the metabolism of monoamine neurotransmitters, particularly noradrenaline (norepinephrine) and serotonin (5-hydroxytryptamine or 5-HT), and their receptors. Their effectiveness has led to the speculation that the biological basis of major mood disorders may be abnormal function of monoamine neurotransmission, but there is little consistent direct evidence for this.

There are three main classes of antidepressants, tricyclic antidepressants, selective serotonin reuptake inhibitors and monoamine oxidase inhibitors.

> **Tricylclic antidepressants are very dangerous in overdose.**
>
> **Selective serotonin reuptake inhibitors are less dangerous, and these should be considered as first-choice antidepressants in adults in most cases.**

Tricyclic antidepressants

Mechanism of action

These drugs inhibit neuronal uptake of 5-HT and noradrenaline, leading to a cascade of secondary changes in monoamine and other neurotransmitter receptors.

Examples

- Amitriptyline hydrochloride
- Imipramine hydrochloride

Example prescription

AMITRIPTYLINE 25 mg p.o. t.i.d.

Indications

- Endogenous depression
- Panic disorders
- Nocturnal enuresis in children
- Neuropathic pain.

Absolute contraindications

- Recent myocardial infarction
- Cardiac arrhythmias
- Severe liver disease.

Relative contraindications

- Cardiac disease
- Glaucoma
- History of urinary retention
- Hypertension
- Porphyria.

Common side effects

- Dry mouth, nausea, constipation, tremor, sweating
- Sedation, blurred vision, confusion, movement disorders, dystonia
- Reduced seizure threshold, convulsions
- Hypotension, dizziness, syncope
- ECG changes, arrhythmias
- Abnormal liver function tests, jaundice
- Blood dyscrasias
- Hyponatraemia.

Significant interactions

- Alcohol causes increased sedation
- Antagonism of antiepileptic drugs.

Selective serotonin reuptake inhibitors

Selective serotonin reuptake inhibitors (SSRIs) selectively inhibit the reuptake of 5-HT, leading to a sustained increase in 5-HT neurotransmission.

Examples

- Citalopram
- Fluoxetine
- Sertraline
- Paroxetine.

Example prescription

PAROXETINE 20 mg p.o. o.d.

Indications

- Depressive illness
- Obsessive-compulsive disorder
- Panic disorders
- Social phobia.

Absolute contraindications

- Manic phase of bipolar disorder
- Patients aged < 18 years (ineffective and increases the risk of suicide)
- Concurrent or recent use of monoamine oxidase inhibitors (MAOIs).

Relative contraindications

- Epilepsy
- Cardiac disease
- Bleeding disorders
- Pregnancy and breast-feeding
- Hepatic and renal disease.

Common side effects

- Gastrointestinal effects: nausea, vomiting, dyspepsia, change in bowel habit
- Hypersensitivity reactions: rash, urticaria, angioedema, arthralgia, myalgia, anaphylaxis

- CNS effects: sedation, dry mouth, anxiety, tremor, sweating, visual disturbance, convulsions
- Endocrine effects: raised prolactin, galactorrhoea, hyponatraemia
- Bleeding disorders
- Cardiovascular effects: palpitations, tachycardia.

Significant interactions

- Sedative effects increased with alcohol
- Antagonism of antiepileptic drug effects
- Increased plasma concentration of antipsychotics
- CNS toxicity with triptans (used in the treatment of migraine)
- CNS excitation with dopaminergic agents, eg selegiline.

Monoamine oxidase inhibitors

Mechanism of action

MAOIs inhibit monoamine oxidase, causing an accumulation of amine neurotransmitters (5-HT, noradrenaline and dopamine). The enzyme also inhibits the metabolism of amine drugs (such as phenylephrine in cold remedies and decongestants) and tyramine in foods (cheese, meat extracts), and in combination with these substances can cause severe hypertensive crises. As a result of these interactions, MAOIs are now rarely, if ever, used in the treatment of depression.

Drugs for migraine

Migraine is a condition characterised by repeated attacks of moderate or severe headache lasting 4–72 hours. The headache is characteristically unilateral, throbbing, aggravated by movement, associated with nausea or vomiting, and accompanied by photophobia and phonophobia. Patients can often identify trigger factors such as too much or too little sleep, skipping meals, changes in stress levels, excessive exercise or changes in afferent stimuli (such as high levels of light). Treatments for migraine aim to:

- Treat the symptoms of the acute attack
- Prevent attacks, in patients whose attacks are frequent and severe enough to consider taking regular preventive treatment.

Essential physiology

Migraine is classified as a neurovascular headache. There is a primary disturbance of brain function in migraine, with vascular changes occurring as secondary phenomena. The headache is thought to be related to dilatation of the intracranial blood vessels, with shunting of blood flow via arteriovenous anastomoses, or alternatively to the release of proinflammatory neuropeptides in the perivascular space.

Treatment of the acute attack of migraine

When nausea and vomiting prevent use of oral medication, many treatments can be administered sublingually, rectally, intranasally or by subcutaneous injection. Therapeutic options include:

- Simple analgesia such as paracetamol (see page 202), with antiemetics (see page 114)
- Non-steroidal anti-inflammatory drugs (NSAIDs, see page 203)
- Triptans
- Ergotamine.

Triptans

Mechanism of action

These drugs are 5-HT$_{1B/1D}$ receptor agonists. They have a low affinity for other subtypes of 5-HT receptors, and are thought to act by causing constriction of intracranial blood vessels, including arteriovenous anastomoses, or by inhibiting neurotransmitter release in the perivascular space.

Examples

- Sumatriptan
- Zolmitriptan
- Naratriptan.

Example prescription

SUMATRIPTAN 100 mg p.o. once only

Indications

- Acute migraine attack
- Cluster headache.

Absolute contraindications

- Ischaemic heart disease
- Severe hypertension.

Relative contraindications

- Previous stroke or transient ischaemic attack
- Peripheral vascular disease.

Common side effects

- Tingling, heat or heaviness in any part of body
- Flushing
- Dizziness, weakness, faintness
- Hypersensitivity: rashes, urticaria, angioedema, anaphylaxis
- Myalgia, muscle weakness
- Drowsiness.

Interactions

- Increased CNS toxicity with antidepressants
- Risk of vasospasm when given with ergotamine.

Ergotamine

Ergotamine is a vasoconstrictor. As a result of its side effects, its use is restricted to those who do not respond to analgesics and triptans. Side effects include nausea, vomiting, abdominal pain and muscular cramps. In overdose it causes ergotism, which is characterised by vasospasm, gangrene of the digits and confusion. It is sometimes used short term, under specialist supervision, for cluster headache, another neurovascular headache syndrome. Cluster headaches usually respond to triptans or 100% oxygen at a rate of 7–12 l/minute.

Prophylaxis of migraine

Prophylactic drugs are indicated if sufferers, having addressed trigger factors, still have frequent severe episodes. A number of drugs are used. In general, about two-thirds of patients can expect a 50% reduction in frequency of episodes with most of these drugs.

Mechanism of action

Many drugs have been used for migraine prophylaxis (Table 6.1). How they work is largely unknown.

Drug name	Dosage	Side effects
Pizotifen	500 micrograms–2 mg daily	Drowsiness, weight gain
Propranolol	40–120 mg b.d.	See page 52
Amitriptyline	25–75 mg nocte	See page 138
Sodium valproate	400–600 mg b.d.	See page 154
Topiramate	25–100 mg	See page 153

Table 6.1 Drugs used in migraine prophylaxis

Anticonvulsants

An epileptic seizure is an abnormal paroxysmal synchronous discharge of neurones which causes disturbances of sensation, movement or consciousness apparent to the patient or onlooker. In all people, seizures can be provoked by stimuli such as chemical convulsants or electroconvulsant therapy (ECT). Epilepsy is a chronic condition where seizures occur without external provocation.

Seizures caused by changes that remain confined to a focal area in the brain are called partial seizures. Those that involve both cerebral hemispheres from the outset are classified as generalised seizures. In simple partial seizures consciousness is preserved, whereas in complex partial seizures there is disturbance of consciousness.

Epilepsy is also classified into various epilepsy syndromes that refer to a cluster of symptoms, including seizure type, age of onset, etc (eg juvenile myoclonic epilepsy).

The aim of anticonvulsant treatment is to prevent recurrence of seizures. Combinations of drugs are used only if monotherapy with several drugs used individually and tried sequentially, has been ineffective. This is because the risks of toxicity and interactions increase with use of multiple drugs. The initial choice of drug depends on the type of seizure or seizure syndrome, as well as patient factors, eg carbamazepine is ineffective in juvenile myoclonic epilepsy and sodium valproate is avoided in young women because of side effects of menstrual disturbance and teratogenicity. Some anticonvulsants (eg phenytoin) have a small therapeutic index, and monitoring of drug levels is needed if toxicity is suspected or if the therapeutic effect is suboptimal. Apart from checking compliance, monitoring blood levels of other anticonvulsants is unhelpful.

Lamogitrine and sodium valproate are commonly used for primary generalised epilepsy. Carbamazepine, lamogitrine and sodium valproate are commonly used in focal epilepsy. Phenotoin is a second line drug and should not be used in young females because of its side effects. Newer anti-epileptic drugs (topiramate, levetiracetam, gabapentin, pregabalin) are, at present, less commonly used as first-line treatment.

The drug chosen as monotherapy should be started at a low dose, and increased slowly either until the seizures remit, or adverse effects emerge.

All antiepileptic drugs carry an inreased risk of teratogenicity, so specialist referral for pre-pregnancy counselling and antenatal screening for neural tube defects if necessary. Patients should take 5 g folic acid daily prior to conception until the end of the first trimester, to reduce the risk of such congenital anomalies.

Essential physiology

The CNS contains high levels of amino acids such as glutamate and GABA, which are highly potent in their ability to alter neuronal discharges. The dicarboxylic amino acids (glutamate, aspartate) produce excitation whereas monocarboxylic amino acids (GABA, glycine, taurine, β alanine) produce inhibition. These neurotransmitters interact with selective receptors on neurones. At a cellular level, the excitability of neurones is achieved through modification of ion channels on plasma membranes. There are sodium, potassium, calcium and chloride channels.

Anticonvulsant drugs achieve their effects by a number of mechanisms:

- Limiting the sustained repetitive firing of a neurone: this effect is mediated by promoting the inactivated state of voltage-activated sodium channels.
- Enhancing GABA-mediated synaptic inhibition: this can be presynaptic for some drugs and postsynaptic for others.
- Inhibiting activation of voltage-activated calcium channels.

Box 6.1 Commonly used antiepileptic drugs	
Carbamazepine	Phenobarbital
Ethosuximide	Phenytoin
Gabapentin and pregabalin	Topiramate
Lamotrigine	Valproate
Levetiracetam	Clonazepam

Carbamazepine

Mechanism of action

Carbamazepine slows the rate of recovery of voltage-activated sodium channels after they have been activated.

Example prescription

TEGRETOL RETARD® 400 mg p.o. b.d.

Indications

- Partial and secondary generalised seizures
- Tonic–clonic seizures
- Trigeminal neuralgia
- Prophylaxis of bipolar disorder unresponsive to lithium.

Absolute contraindications

- Cardiac conduction abnormalities.

Relative contraindications

- Liver impairment
- Cardiac disease.

Common side effects

- Nausea and vomiting
- Dizziness, ataxia
- Confusion, agitation

- Generalised rash or photosensitive rash
- Blood disorders including marrow depression
- Jaundice
- Hyponatraemia
- Galactorrhoea.

Significant interactions

Carbamazepine is an inducer of liver enzymes, and can therefore enhance the metabolism of other drugs (see page 12).

Ethosuximide

Mechanism of action

Ethosuximide reduces low-threshold calcium currents in thalamic neurones.

Example prescription

ETHOSUXIMIDE 500 mg p.o b.d.

Indications

- Simple absence seizures
- Myoclonic seizures
- Atypical absence, atonic and tonic seizures.

Absolute contraindication

Porphyria.

Relative contraindication

Impairment of liver or renal function.

Common side effects

- Gastrointestinal tract disturbances
- Hepatic and renal dysfunction
- Drowsiness, ataxia, dystonia, hiccup
- Blood dyscrasias (rarely).

Significant interactions

The antiepileptic effect is reduced by phenytoin, carbamazepine, antidepressants and antipsychotics.

Gabapentin

Mechanism of action

Gabapentin was developed to be a centrally acting GABA agonist. It is highly lipid soluble. The molecular structure of gabapentin is that of a GABA molecule covalently bound to a cyclohexane ring. However, the mechanism of the anticonvulsant effect of gabapentin is unknown. Gabapentin has not been found to reduce sustained repetitive firing of action potentials.

Example prescription

GABAPENTIN 300 mg p.o. b.d.

Indications

- Adjunctive treatment in partial seizures
- Neuropathic pain.

Relative contraindication

History of psychiatric illness.

Common side effects

- Dry mouth, dyspepsia, nausea and vomiting
- Dizziness, nystagmus, tremor
- Weight gain
- Peripheral oedema.

Significant interactions

The anticonvulsant effect is reduced by antidepressants.

Pregabalin

Pregabalin is a precursor of gabapentin, and has similar indications. It has fewer side effects than gabapentin.

Lamotrigine

Mechanism of action

Lamotrigine delays the recovery from inactivation of recombinant Na^+ channels and may also inhibit synaptic release of glutamate by acting at Na^+ channels.

Example prescription

LAMOTRIGINE 100 mg p.o b.d.

Indications

- Partial seizures
- Primary and secondary generalised tonic-clonic seizures.

Contraindications

Caution with liver, haematological and renal disease.

Common side effects

- Rashes, including Stevens–Johnson syndrome; the risk is reduced by slowly titrating the dose, and increased by combining the drug with valproate
- Drowsiness, headache, ataxia, agitation, confusion
- Blood disorders
- Angioedema.

Significant interactions

- Its effect is reduced by antidepressants.
- The plasma concentration is increased by valproate.
- The plasma concentration is reduced by enzyme-inducing anticonvulsants (eg carbamazepine, phenytoin).

Levetiracetam

Mechanism of action
The mechanism of action is unknown.

Example prescription
LEVETIRACETAM 500 mg p.o. b.d.

Indication
Adjunctive treatment of partial seizures.

Contraindication
Liver impairment.

Common side effects
- Drowsiness, dizziness, ataxia, vertigo
- Mood disturbance
- Blood dyscrasias.

Phenobarbital

Mechanism of action
Phenobarbital potentiates synaptic inhibition by acting on GABA receptors. At high levels, phenobarbital also limits repetitive neuronal firing.

Example prescription
PHENOBARBITAL 120 mg p.o. nocte

Indications
- Partial seizures
- Primary and secondary generalised tonic-clonic seizures
- Status epilepticus.

Contraindications
Hepatic impairment, renal impairment, porphyria.

Common side effects

- Sedation, drowsiness, lethargy
- Depression, confusion, restlessness
- Megaloblastic anaemia
- Exfoliative dermatitis.

Significant interactions

- The plasma concentration of phenobarbital is increased by valproate.
- There is an increased sedative effect with alcohol.
- There is increased metabolism of various drugs, leading to reduced therapeutic effects (see page 12).

Phenytoin

Phenytoin has a non-linear dose–response curve and a narrow therapeutic index. This means that small changes in its dose can cause large changes in plasma concentration and subsequently toxic side effects can occur. Monitoring plasma concentration is therefore very helpful in dosage adjustment. The optimum therapeutic concentration is 10–20 mg/l.

Mechanism of action

Phenytoin slows the rate of recovery of voltage-activated Na^+ channels after they are inactivated.

Example prescription

EPANUTIN® 300 mg p.o. nocte.

Phenytoin preparations vary in their bioavailability, so are not interchangeable. It is always necessary to specify the proprietary name when prescribing.

Indications

- Status epilepticus
- Tonic-clonic seizures
- Partial seizures.

Absolute contraindication

Porphyria.

Relative contraindications

- Hepatic impairment
- Breast-feeding.

Common side effects

- Gum hypertrophy
- Gingival hyperplasia
- Nausea, vomiting
- Dizziness, headache, tremor, confusion
- Blood dyscrasias, including agranulocytosis
- Stevens–Johnson syndrome
- Osteomalacia
- Ataxia, blurred vision, nystagmus and slurred speech are signs of overdosage.

Significant interactions

Phenytoin is an inducer of liver enzymes and therefore can affect the metabolism of many drugs metabolised in the liver (see page 12):

- May reduce anticoagulant effect of warfarin.
- Reduced plasma concentration of carbamazepine, lamogitrine, topiramate and valproate.
- Its anticonvulsant effect is antagonised by antipsychotics and SSRIs
- Phenytoin accelerates the metabolism of oestrogens and progesterone; the oral contraceptive pill will therefore have reduced contraceptive effect.
- Neurotoxicity when given with lithium (can occur without increased plasma concentration of lithium).

Topiramate

Mechanism of action

Topiramate has a range of anti-seizure actions. It reduces voltage-gated sodium currents, enhances postsynaptic GABA receptor currents and limits activation of some subtypes of glutamate receptor.

Example prescription

SODIUM VALPROATE 50 mg p.o. b.d.

Indications

- Tonic-clonic seizures
- Partial seizures.

Absolute contraindication

Porphyria.

Relative contraindications

Hepatic and renal impairment.

Common side effects

- Nausea, abdominal pain, weight loss, anorexia
- Drowsiness, fatigue.

Significant interactions

- The anticonvulsant effect is antagonised by SSRIs and tricyclic antidepressants.
- Accelerated metabolism of oestrogen and progesterone, reducing the efficacy of oral contraceptives.

Valproate

Mechanism of action

Valproate inhibits sustained prolonged repetitive firing by prolonging recovery of voltage-activated Na^+ channels after they are inactivated.

Example prescription

EPILIM CHRONO® 600 mg p.o. b.d.

Indication

All forms of epilepsy.

Absolute contraindications

- Active liver disease
- Porphyria.

Relative contraindications

- Pregnancy
- Renal impairment
- Systemic lupus erythematosus.

Common side effects

- Increased appetite and weight gain
- Tremor
- Menstrual disturbance and polycystic ovarian syndrome
- Jaundice and liver impairment
- Rashes
- Pancreatitis
- Blood dyscrasias.

Drug interactions

- Anticonvulsant effects antagonised by antipsychotics and antidepressants
- Plasma concentration of valproate reduced by carbamazepine
- Valproate increases plasma level of lamotrigine.

Clonazepam

Clonazepam is a benzodiazepine occasionally used as adjunctive treatment in tonic-clonic or partial seizures, but its use is limited by its sedative side effects. See page 132 for more information on benzodiazepines.

Mood-stabilising drugs

Lithium is used in the prophylaxis and treatment of manic-depressive illness (also known as 'bipolar disorder').

Mechanism of action

Lithium salts have effects on receptor transduction systems, including the turnover of phosphoinositols, that may prevent excessive intracellular signalling. Lithium also increases brain 5-HT function. Lithium has a therapeutic index and its excretion is critically dependent on the kidneys. Plasma levels and renal function should always be monitored in patients treated with lithium salts.

Examples

- Lithium carbonate
- Lithium citrate.

Example prescription

PRIADEL® 800 mg p.o. o.d.

Lithium preparations vary widely in bioavailability, so they are not prescribed generically.

Indications

- Treatment and prophylaxis of bipolar disorder
- Prophylaxis of cluster headache.

Absolute contraindication

Renal failure.

Relative contraindications

- Any disorder causing abnormal fluid and electrolyte balance
- Renal impairment.

Common side effects

- Tremor
- Nausea
- Thirst and polyuria (resulting from nephrogenic diabetes insipidus)
- Hypothyroidism
- Toxic levels (> 2.0 mmol/l) cause drowsiness, dysarthria, seizures, coma, renal failure and cardiovascular collapse.

Significant interactions

- Thiazide diuretics and NSAIDs can cause lithium toxicity.
- Increased risk of extrapyramidal movement disorders when antipsychotic drugs are used concomitantly.

Drugs for Parkinson's disease and other movement disorders

Essential physiology

Parkinson's disease is a neurodegenerative disorder characterised by progressive and irreversible loss of dopaminergic neurones in the substantia nigra (one of the basal ganglia), resulting in a disorder of movement. Typically, there is tremor, rigidity, bradykinesia and impairment of balance. Therapies for Parkinson's disease do not alter the course of the disease, but are often effective in treating the symptoms. Parkinsonism, ie the clinical features of Parkinson's disease resulting from other causes such as stroke or antipsychotic drugs, do not respond to dopaminergic drugs, but may respond to antimuscarinic drug therapy (see page 161).

Drugs for Parkinson's disease and parkinsonism

Dopaminergic drugs

Four types of dopaminergic drugs are used in Parkinson's disease:

1. Dopamine receptor agonists
2. Levodopa
3. Monoamine oxidase-B (MAO-B) inhibitors
4. Catechol-O-methyltransferase (COMT) inhibitors.

Dopamine receptor agonists

Mechanism of action

Dopamine receptor agonists have direct effects on striatal dopamine receptors. Unlike levodopa, they do not depend on the functional capacity of the nigrostriatal nerves and therefore they may be more effective than levodopa in late Parkinson's disease.

Examples

- Bromocriptine
- Cabergoline
- Lisuride
- Pergolide
- Ropinirole
- Pramipexole.

Example prescription

PERGOLIDE 500 micrograms p.o. t.i.d.

Absolute contraindications

- History of fibrotic disease
- Cardiac valve disease.

Relative contraindications

- Arrhythmias
- Pregnancy and breast-feeding
- Confusion and hallucinations.

Common side effects

- Confusion, hallucinations, drowsiness, diplopia, neuroleptic malignant syndrome (see page 136)
- Hypotension, syncope, tachycardia
- Fibrotic reactions are well recognised but uncommon; pulmonary, cardiac valvular, retroperitoneal and pericardial fibrotic reactions may occur
- Pleuritis, pleural effusion
- Rash, fever, Raynaud's phenomenon.

Significant interactions

The effects of pergolide are antagonised by antipsychotics and metoclopramide.

Levodopa

Mechanism of action

Levodopa is the metabolic precursor of dopamine. Its therapeutic and adverse effects on the CNS result from the decarboxylation of levodopa within pre-synaptic terminals of dopaminergic neurons in the striatum. After release, dopamine is either transported back into dopaminergic terminals or metabolised by the action of the enzymes MAO or COMT.

Levodopa is usually administered in combination with a peripherally acting decarboxylase inhibitor such as carbidopa or benserazide. This markedly reduces the peripheral conversion of levodopa to dopamine, thus limiting the side effects of nausea, vomiting and cardiovascular effects, while allowing effective dopamine concentrations to be achieved in the brain.

Examples

- Madopar®
- Sinemet®.

Example prescription

SINEMET CR® 50/200 mg 1 tablet p.o. b.d.

(This comprises 50 mg carbidopa + 200 mg levodopa per tablet.)

Indication

Parkinson's disease.

Absolute contraindications

- Pregnancy and breast-feeding
- Glaucoma.

Relative contraindications

- Severe psychotic illness
- Peptic ulceration.

Common side effects

- Confusion
- Sudden daytime sleepiness
- Anorexia, nausea, vomiting
- Postural hypotension, tachycardia, arrhythmias
- Psychosis
- Dyskinesia.

Significant interactions

- Hypertensive crisis with MAOI antidepressants
- Enhanced hypotensive effect of all antihypertensives
- Effects of levodopa are antagonised by antipsychotics.

MAO-B inhibitors

Selegiline is used early in the course of Parkinson's disease, delaying the need for levodopa. It can also be used late in the disease when the side effects of levodopa become troublesome.

Mechanism of action

Selegiline is an inhibitor of MAO B, which is responsible for most of the oxidative metabolism of dopamine in the striatum. Unlike non-specific MAOIs, selegiline does not inhibit the peripheral metabolism of catecholamines, and there is therefore no risk of hypertensive crises when tyramine-rich foods are eaten.

Example prescription

SELEGILINE HYDROCHLORIDE 10 mg p.o. b.d.

Absolute contraindications

- Pregnancy, breast-feeding
- Glaucoma.

Relative contraindications

- Cardiovascular disease
- Kidney and liver disease.

Common side effects

- Nausea
- Confusion, hallucinations, agitation
- Postural hypotension
- Headache.

Significant interactions

- CNS toxicity and fever with opiates
- CNS system excitation with antidepressants
- Enhances effects and toxicity of other dopaminergics

COMT inhibitors

Mechanism of action

These drugs block the catabolism of levodopa and dopamine, increasing the plasma half-life of levodopa and the amount of each administered dose that reaches the CNS. They are used in combination with levodopa/carbidopa under specialist supervision.

Examples

- Entacapone
- Tolcapone.

Example prescription

TOLCAPONE 100 mg p.o. t.i.d.

Absolute contraindications

- Liver disease
- Dyskinesia

Relative contraindications

Pregnancy and breast-feeding.

Common side effects

- Hepatotoxicity (potentially life-threatening)
- Nausea and vomiting
- Orthostatic hypotension
- Confusion, vivid dreams, hallucinations.

Significant interactions

- Avoid use with MAOI antidepressants

Anti-muscarinic drugs

Mechanism of action

As a result of dopamine deficiency, there is central cholinergic excess. Anti-muscarinic drugs reduce the effects of this excess. These drugs are not used in Parkinson's disease because dopaminergic drugs are more effective, although they are used in parkinsonism from other causes, where dopaminergic drugs are ineffective.

Examples

- Benzatropine
- Orphenadrine
- Procyclidine.

Example prescription

BENZATROPINE MESILATE 1 mg p.o. nocte

Indications

- Drug-induced parkinsonism
- Emergency treatment of acute drug-induced dystonic reactions (but ineffective for tardive dyskinesia).

Absolute contraindication

Gastrointestinal tract obstruction.

Relative contraindications

- Cardiovascular disease
- Prostatic hypertrophy
- Hepatic and renal impairment
- Pregnancy and breast-feeding.

Common side effects

- Constipation, nausea, vomiting
- Agitation, confusion, hallucinations, restlessness, insomnia
- Urinary retention.

Drug interactions

Use of two or more antimuscarinic drugs can increase side effects.

Other drugs used for movement disorders

These are all used under specialist supervision:

- Riluzole is used in the amyotrophic lateral sclerosis form of motor neuron disease. It has modest effects in delaying disability.
- Tetrabenazine is used in Huntington's disease.
- Botulinum toxin is injected locally for muscle spasticity in a number of conditions, eg blepharospasm
- Beta-blockers (non-cardioselective) are used for essential tremor.

Drugs for vertigo

Vertigo is the subjective sensation of movement. It is usually described as a feeling of rotation, but sometimes comprises a feeling of side-to-side motion. Often there is associated nausea and vomiting and difficulty with balance. Vertigo is caused by problems in the brainstem or within the vestibular nerve or semi-circular canals of the inner ear.

There is no effective prophylactic treatment for vertigo so long-term therapy is not indicated. For severe attacks, drugs that act as vestibular sedatives can be used, but only for the duration of the attack.

Phenothiazines

These drugs should not be used long term for non-specific dizziness in elderly people, because vestibular sedation may make problems with balance worse. See page 135 for further details.

Mechanism of action

These drugs are dopamine antagonists, and act centrally by blockade of the chemoreceptor trigger zone.

Example prescription

PROCHLORPERAZINE 5mg p.o. t.i.d.

Antihistamines

These agents are used principally for motion sickness and as antiemetics. They can be taken prophylactically. They vary in their duration of action and side-effect profile (principally the degree of sedation and anti-muscarinic side effects). See pages 115 and 246 for details.

Examples

- Cinnarazine
- Cyclizine
- Promethazine.

Example prescription

PROMETHAZINE 25 mg p.o. 1–2 hours before travel for motion sickness

Betahistine

Mechanism of action

This is an analogue of histamine, and it is thought to reduce endolymphatic pressure in the inner ear by improving microcirculation.

Example prescription

BETAHISTINE 16 mg p.o. t.i.d.

Indication

Ménière's disease.

Absolute contraindication

Phaeochromocytoma.

Relative contraindications

- Asthma
- Peptic ulcer disease
- Pregnancy and breast-feeding.

Common side effects

- Gastrointestinal tract disturbances
- Headache
- Rashes and itch.

Significant interactions

None of note.

Management of acute alcohol withdrawal and delirium tremens

Alcohol withdrawal symptoms usually occur within 24 hours of admission to hospital. Of course, the onset of symptoms will depend on when the patient last drank alcohol. The condition is entially serious. If a patient progresses to delirium tremens, mortality approaches 20%. Complications such as liver failure, hypoglycaemia and subarachnoid haemorrhage can occur.

SYMPTOMS AND SIGNS OF ALCOHOL WITHDRAWAL

EARLY	Mild acute tremulousness of head, hands, legs, trunk
	Nausea, retching, sweating
	Misperceptions, hallucinations (24–48hrs)
	Agitation 'must leave hospital', insomnia
	Disorientation in time and place
	Clouding of consciousness, impairment of recent memory
LATE	Autonomic Disturbance (fever, tachycardia, blood pressure)
SEVERE	Seizures (after 7–48 hours)

DROWSINESS IS NOT A FEATURE OF ALCOHOL WITHDRAWAL.
OTHER CAUSES SHOULD BE CONSIDERED

Where appropriate, patients should be nursed in an area with adequate lighting.

Ideally, delirium tremens (DTs) should be pre-empted rather than waiting for it to develop. Consider treatment with benzodiazepines when there are:

- Moderate to severe signs and symptoms of withdrawal
- Mild symptoms with risk factors for progression to severe withdrawal and DTs: if drinking more than 15 units/day, a history of previous DTs or severe withdrawal/seizures, other psychotropic drugs, poor physical and mental health, high levels of anxiety, low glucose, potassium or calcium, fever, sweating, insomnia and tachycardia.

Be wary of dehydration, hypoglycaemia and delirium caused by an infection or head injury.

Benzodiazepines are the drugs of choice for alcohol withdrawal. The particular drug used depends on the presence or absence of significant liver impairment. Chlordiazepoxide is used if there is no significant liver disease. No fixed dosage schedule will meet all situations. Lower doses than those suggested may be used in elderly people, women and those with respiratory disease. Hypotension, respiratory depression and sedation are signs of excessive dosing. The dose and choice of benzodiazepine should be reviewed in the presence of these symptoms (Table 6.2).

Day		Chlordiazepoxide dose
1	Regular	20–40 mg q.i.d.
	p.r.n.	20–30 mg 2- to 4-hourly p.r.n.
	Daily maximum dose	320 mg in 24 hours
2		20–40 mg q.i.d.
3		10–20 mg t.i.d.
4		10–20 mg t.i.d.
5		10–20 mg t.i.d.
6		10 mg b.d.
7		10 mg b.d.

Adapted with permission from a protocol developed by Dr Judith O'Neill (Consultant Psychiatrist) and Carmel Darcy (Pharmacist), Causeway Hospital, Coleraine, Northern Ireland.

Table 6.2 Dose of chlordiazepoxide used in the treatment of delirium tremens

Nursing staff should omit the prescribed dose if the patient is over-sedated.

Intravenous diazepam is an alternative to chlordiazepoxide in very agitated patients unable to take oral treatment. Diazemuls® 10 mg should be given intravenously over 2 minutes. The dose can be repeated after 4 hours if there is no improvement.

Seizures

Adequate doses of chlordiazepoxide usually prevent withdrawal seizures. For isolated seizures, continue with the standard regimen, ensuring that the patient has received an adequate dose. If a patient develops prolonged or recurrent seizures give lorazepam 2 mg i.v. as a single dose (in addition to existing benzodiazepines). If fitting continues, seek senior advice.

Hallucinations/delusions

Haloperidol 1.5–5 mg p.o. or i.m. two to three times daily (maximum 30 mg/24 hours) can be used with caution and in the short term. It has epileptogenic potential.

Vitamin prophylaxis

All patients should have thiamine supplements orally or intravenously, depending on their clinical state as shown below.

> **Never forget**
>
> All alcohol-dependent patients should be given B vitamins intravenously before treatment with intravenous glucose.
>
> This is because glucose can precipitate Wernicke's encephalopathy in patients deficient in B vitamins.

Confirmed or imminent Wernicke's encephalopathy

Give vitamins B and C (Pabrinex®), two pairs of ampoules three times daily by intravenous infusion for 3 days, followed by one pair once daily for 3–5 days or until clinical improvement occurs. Then switch to oral thiamine as below.

Patients at risk of Wernicke's encephalopathy

This includes patients with significant weight loss, poor diet or signs of malnutrition.

Give vitamins B and C (Pabrinex®), one pair of ampoules once daily by intravenous infusion for 3 days, then switch to oral thiamine as below.

Uncomplicated alcohol withdrawal

Oral vitamins should be prescribed as follows: vitamin B compound (strong) one tablet daily and 300 mg thiamine daily. Supplementation should be continued long term.

Treatment regimen at discharge

Patients started on the above benzodiazepine withdrawal regimens should be discharged on an appropriate reducing regimen. All patients should be discharged on the recommended vitamins. Ensure that advice has been given about services available to help with overcoming alcohol dependence.

Note that relatively short-acting benzodiazepines (eg lorazepam) have a high addictive potential and should not be prescribed at discharge.

Management of status epilepticus

The fundamental goal of treatment is to stop seizure activity immediately. General measures should be considered alongside specific anticonvulsant therapy. A patient still convulsing within 30 minutes of admission should be admitted to intensive care for management.

General measures and investigations

See Table 6.3 for these.

First stage (0–10 minutes)	Airway management, with high-flow oxygen (100%) Intravenous access and cardiovascular resuscitation
Second stage (0–60 minutes)	Initiate emergency drug therapy (see below) Intravenous glucose and thiamine Monitoring of vital signs (temperature, pulse, blood pressure and respiratory rate) Monitoring neurological signs (Glasgow Coma Score, lateralising signs, pupils) O_2 saturation monitoring and acid–base balance (ABG analysis required) Blood tests (U&Es, LFTs, Ca^{2+}, Mg^{2+}, glucose), FBC Anticonvulsant levels to assess compliance with prior prescriptions (available only for phenytoin, carbamazepine and sodium valproate)
Third stage (up to 60 minutes)	Establish cause: CT of brain (must not compromise patient vital signs) Correct physiological abnormalities (pulse, blood pressure, biochemistry) Consider inotropes
Fourth stage (30–90 minutes)	Intensive care admission Invasive monitoring EEG at next available opportunity Initiate maintenance anticonvulsants Discuss with neurologist Raised intracranial pressure management may require discussion with neurosurgery

ABG, arterial blood gas; CT, computed tomography; EEG, electroencephalograph; FBC, full blood count; LFTs, liver function tests; U&Es, urea and electrolytes.
From M Walker and S Shorvon (2005) *ILAE Epilepsy Course Book*, St Anne's College, Oxford.

Table 6.3 General measures and investigations for management of status epilepticus

Drug therapy

Benzodiazepines are the preferred agents for initial therapy. The two most commonly used are diazepam and lorazepam. They are equally effective in stopping seizures but lorazepam has a much longer duration of anti-seizure effect than diazepam (12–24 hours compared with 15–30 minutes) and is therefore the preferred benzodiazepine for the initial treatment of status epilepticus.

If seizure activity persists after treatment with a benzodiazepine, a second drug needs to be given. Phenytoin should be given as a loading dose. The loading dose is mixed with 0.9% saline, and should be infused at a rate no greater then 50 mg/minute through a wide-bore intravenous cannula. ECG and blood pressure monitoring are required when phenytoin is infused, and the infusion must run through a microfilter. Note that phenytoin should always be made up with saline and used immediately; it should not be stored in this form. Once the loading dose is given, maintenance therapy is continued with an oral or intravenous daily dose of 5–6 mg/kg, guided by blood levels. Fosphenytoin is a water-soluble pro-drug of phenytoin. It can be given more quickly than phenytoin (up to 150 mg phenytoin equivalents/minute). It is also less likely to cause phlebitis.

Box 6.2 Intravenous phenytoin therapy

Always reconstitute phenytoin with 0.9% saline immediately before use

Attach a microfilter to the giving set

Only give through a large-bore intravenous cannula

Monitor blood pressure and the ECG during the infusion

If the patient has not responded to benzodiazepine and phenytoin, admission to an intensive care unit is needed because the next drug of choice is phenobarbital, which depresses the respiratory drive, level of consciousness and blood pressure. If status epilepticus becomes refractory, infusion of anaesthetic doses of midazolam, barbiturates or propofol is needed, together with ventilatory and cardiovascular support (Table 6.4).

Stage	Treatment
Premonitory stage (usually pre-hospital)	Diazepam 10 mg rectally or midazalom 10 mg bucally (repeat after 15 minutes if needed)
Early (on admission – 10 minutes)	Lorazepam 0.07 mg/kg i.v. (usually 4–8 mg bolus) (repeat once after 10 minutes)
Established (10–30 minutes)	Phenytoin 15 mg/kg i.v. at 50 mg/min or fosphenytoin 15 mg PE at 150 mg PE /minute
Refractory (treatment in ICU setting) (> 30 minutes)	Phenobarbital 10 mg/kg at 100 mg/minute (usually 700 mg over 7 minutes). Then, if still seizing 30 min from onset, propofol, midazalom or thiopental general anaesthesia

ICU, intensive care unit; PE, phenytoin equivalent.
Table 6.4 Treatment for status epilepticus

Maintenance anticonvulsants

Long-term maintenance anticonvulsants should be administered along with any treatment for status epilepticus. This includes any prescribed anticonvulsant medication before admission. In addition, phenytoin should be administered as a maintenance dose, following on from any intravenous loading dose. If necessary, administer anticonvulsants via a nasogastric tube. Inadvertent omission of anticonvulsants can increase the risk of recurrent seizures.

Bibliography

Bazire S. *Psychotropic Drug Directory: The professionals' pocket handbook and aide memoire*, 10th edn. Salisbury: Fivepin Publishing Ltd, 2003.

British National Formulary. No 46. London: Pharmaceutical Press, 2003.

Electronic Medicines Compendium, 2004 (http://emc.medicines.org.uk/)

Link Pharmaceuticals. *Trust Protocol: The management of the alcohol withdrawal syndrome and Wernicke's encephalopathy*, 2002.

Royal College of Physicians. *Alcohol – can the NHS afford it?* London: Royal College of Physicians of London, 2001.

Thomson AD et al. *Alcohol and Alcoholism* 2002; **37**: 513–21.

7
Endocrine system

7
Endocrine system

Insulin

Essential physiology and mode of action

Diabetes mellitus is characterised by chronic hyperglycaemia. It is the result of deficiency of insulin, resistance to insulin action or a combination of the two.

Insulin is a polypeptide hormone of central importance in carbohydrate, fat and protein metabolism. It acts by binding to receptors in insulin-sensitive tissues such as the liver, muscle, fat and brain, and promotes glycogen synthesis, protein synthesis and peripheral glucose uptake, while reducing lipolysis and gluconeogenesis. Insulin lowers the levels of glucose, fatty acids, ketone bodies and amino acids in the blood. A mild degree of insulin deficiency disturbs carbohydrate metabolism, giving rise to glycosuria and thirst. Moderate insulin deficiency will, in addition, cause disturbances of protein metabolism, giving rise to weight loss. Severe insulin deficiency will also cause ketosis and life-threatening acidosis.

Type 1 diabetes results from a lack of insulin, and is caused by autoimmune destruction of insulin-producing pancreatic islet β cells. Type 1 diabetes requires treatment with insulin.

As insulin would be digested if taken orally, it has to be given by injection. The injection is usually subcutaneous, but in special circumstances it can be given intravenously or intramuscularly. In the past, insulins extracted from pork and beef pancreas were widely used, but most insulins in current use are produced by recombinant DNA technology, and have the same sequence of amino acids as human insulin. Human insulin analogues have been produced in which a change in the amino acid sequence of the insulin confers different pharmacokinetic properties such as a faster or slower onset of action. These new insulins are increasingly used in basal bolus insulin regimens.

Types of insulin

There are three main types of insulin:

1. Those with a rapid onset of action, such as soluble insulin, insulin aspart and insulin lispro (proprietary names Actrapid®, Humalog® and Novorapid®).

2. Those with an intermediate duration of action, such as isophane insulin (proprietary name Insulatard®).

3. Those with a slow onset and long duration of action, such as insulin glargine, insulin detemir and insulin zinc suspension (proprietary names Lantus®, Levemir® and Ultratard®).

The choice of insulin type and the combinations of insulin used (the insulin regimen) depend on the individual patient. Most newly diagnosed patients are now started on short-acting insulin three times daily before main meals, with an intermediate- or long-acting insulin at bedtime. Some patients can be well controlled on a twice-daily mixture of short- and intermediate-acting insulin, taken before breakfast and before the evening meal. All insulins in current use are of a standard concentration – 100 units/ml. Insulin can be drawn up from vials using specially designed insulin syringes (0.5 or 1 ml). Increasingly, pen devices are used: these contain insulin stored in cartridges, and have the advantage of convenience and the facility for the patient to 'dial the dose'. Another method of delivery is continuous subcutaneous insulin infusion using a portable pump device. This allows the continuous delivery of a basal dose of insulin and there is a patient-controlled bolus of insulin that is delivered at meal times.

> When insulin is prescribed, the word 'units' must be written in full to avoid errors (eg 3 units written as 3U could be mistaken for 30 units).

Insulin dosages

The daily requirement of insulin for patients who are not obese is, on average, 0.5 unit/kg per day. However, if the body mass index (BMI) is > 30, more than 1 unit/kg per day may be needed. Insulin doses are adjusted to maintain blood glucose as close as possible to the normal range.

Insulin requirements may increase significantly in severe acute illnesses such as infection and trauma. This results from high circulating levels of anti-insulin hormones such as corticosteroids and catecholamines. Steroids used therapeutically will also cause a marked increase in blood glucose. The prognosis for patients who have diabetes and are ill for other reasons (eg severe sepsis or acute myocardial infarction) is improved by maintaining excellent glycaemic control. In these circumstances temporary insulin treatment may be needed by patients with type 2 diabetes.

Example prescriptions

> NOVORAPID® 10 units s.c. before breakfast, 6 units s.c. before lunch, 12 units s.c. before evening meal. LANTUS® 24 units s.c. at bedtime

> NOVOMIX 30® 20 units s.c. before breakfast, 12 units s.c. before evening meal

Indications

- Type 1 diabetes
- Type 2 diabetes
- Acute hyperglycaemia and ketoacidosis
- Treatment of hyperkalaemia.

Absolute contraindication

Hypoglycaemia.

Relative contraindication

Dose should be reduced in renal failure.

Common side effects

- Overdose causes hypoglycaemia
- Fat hypertrophy and local reactions at injection sites.

Significant interactions

- Hypoglycaemic effect of insulin is enhanced by alcohol.
- Beta blockers may mask the symptoms of hypoglycaemia.
- Corticosteroids antagonise the effects of insulin.

Oral anti-diabetic drugs

Essential mellitus

Type 2 diabetes is caused by a combination of insulin resistance and insulin deficiency. Most people with type 2 diabetes are obese at diagnosis. Obesity causes insulin resistance, but with increased duration of type 2 diabetes there is a progressive defect of insulin secretion, and eventually some patients with type 2 diabetes will require insulin treatment to control hyperglycaemia. Oral anti-diabetic drugs are prescribed for type 2 diabetes when 3 months of treatment with diet and exercise have failed to improve glycaemic control. Oral hypoglycaemic drugs are often used in combination, and metformin is often prescribed with insulin in type 2 diabetes.

Sulphonylureas

Mechanism of action

These drugs act by stimulating insulin secretion. As a first-line treatment for type 2 diabetes, they are valuable in the minority of patients who are not overweight.

Examples

- Gliclazide
- Glibenclamide
- Glimepiride.

Example prescription

GLICLAZIDE 80 mg p.o. b.d.

Indication

Type 2 diabetes.

Absolute contraindications

- Hypoglycaemia
- Pregnancy.

Relative contraindications

These drugs should be used with caution in renal impairment.

Common side effects

- Hypoglycaemia: all sulphonylureas can cause hypoglycaemia, which can be particularly troublesome in elderly people. It is therefore best to avoid long-acting sulphonylureas (eg glibenclamide) in elderly people. Shorter-acting sulphonylureas (eg gliclazide) are preferable.
- Minor gastrointestinal upsets
- Rashes
- Liver function test (LFT) abnormalities.

Significant interactions

- Alcohol enhances the hypoglycaemic effect of sulphonylureas.
- Corticosteroids antagonise the effect of sulphonylureas.

Biguanides

Mechanism of action

Biguanides act by decreasing gluconeogenesis and increasing peripheral utilisation of glucose. The only biguanide in use is metformin. It should be the first choice of oral hypoglycaemic in the overweight person with type 2 diabetes.

Example

Metformin.

Example prescription

METFORMIN 500 mg p.o. t.i.d.

Indications

- Type 2 diabetes
- Polycystic ovarian syndrome.

Absolute contraindications

- Hypoglycaemia
- Renal failure
- Ketoacidosis
- Pregnancy.

Relative contraindications

Metformin should be stopped in conditions where tissue hypoxia occurs, eg sepsis, myocardial infarction, hepatic impairment, and before intravenous contrast media are used. This is because of the risk of lactic acidosis.

Common side effects

- Anorexia, nausea and vomiting
- Abdominal pain
- Diarrhoea
- Vitamin B_{12} malabsorption.

Thiazolidinediones (glitazones)

These are the most recently developed drugs for type 2 diabetes. When used alone, they are slower to improve blood glucose than either sulphonylureas or metformin. They are often used in combination with metformin, or in place of metformin in combination with sulphonylureas, when patients cannot tolerate metformin.

Mechanism of action

The thiazolidinediones reduce peripheral insulin resistance.

Examples

- Rosiglitazone
- Pioglitazone
- Avandamet® (combination of metformin and rosiglitazone).

Example prescription

ROSIGLITAZONE 8 mg p.o. o.d.

Indication

Type 2 diabetes.

Absolute contraindications

- Hypoglycaemia
- Heart failure
- Pregnancy
- Hepatic impairment.

Relative contraindication

Renal impairment.

Common side effects

- Ankle swelling
- Gastrointestinal tract disturbance
- Weight gain.

Thyroid hormones

Essential physiology

Thyroid hormones are critical for brain and somatic development in infants, and for metabolic activity at all ages. There are large stores of thyroid hormone in the circulation and in the thyroid gland, and thyroid hormone biosynthesis and secretion are regulated by mechanisms that are very sensitive to slight changes in circulating hormone concentrations.

The thyroid is composed of follicles, each comprising a single layer of follicular cells surrounding a lumen filled with colloid, mostly thyroglobulin. When stimulated, the follicular cells change shape, becoming columnar, and the lumen is depleted of colloid.

There are two thyroid hormones: thyroxine (T_4), which contains four iodine atoms, and triiodothyronine (T_3), which has three. T_4 is produced solely by thyroid tissue and most of the T_3 is produced in extrathyroidal tissues by deiodination of T_4. T_4 and T_3 are both synthesised and stored in the thyroid gland, incorporated in thyroglobulin.

Iodine is essential for normal thyroid function. It is transported as iodide into follicular cells, where it is oxidised in a reaction catalysed by thyroid peroxidase. It is then bound covalently to tyrosyl residues of thyroglobulin. Coupling of two diiodotyrosine residues produces T_4, whereas coupling of one diiodotyrosine residue and one monoiodotyrosine residue produces T_3. These reactions are also catalysed by thyroid peroxidase.

Over 99% of T_4 and T_3 in the serum is bound to protein, so changes in the concentration of binding proteins can have a major effect on the serum T_4 and T_3, but not on the biologically active free T_4 and T_3. Modern assays measure free hormones.

Thyroid hormone production is regulated by thyroid-stimulating hormone (TSH) secreted by the anterior pituitary gland. Secretion of TSH is inhibited by T_4 and T_3, and stimulated by thyrotrophin-releasing hormone (TRH), secreted from the hypothalamus. TSH stimulates all stages of thyroid hormone synthesis and secretion, and promotes thyroid growth.

T_3 and T_4

Mechanism of action

T_4 and T_3 enter cells by diffusion. T_4 is converted to T_3, which then binds to nuclear receptors and affects the function of every organ system.

Examples

- Levothyroxine sodium (T_4) is the commonly used thyroid hormone.
- Liothyronine sodium (T_3) is used in myxoedema coma, because it has a more rapid onset of action than T_4.

Example prescription

LEVOTHYROXINE 100 micrograms p.o o.d.

Standard dosages

The usual starting dose is 50–100 micrograms daily, adjusted in steps of 50 micrograms every 4–6 weeks until the patient is biochemically (TSH normal) and clinically euthyroid. Smaller starting doses are used in patients who have ischaemic heart disease.

Indications

- Primary hypothyroidism
- Secondary hypothyroidism
- Post-radioactive-iodine hypothyroidism
- Thyroid cancer.

Contraindication

Thyrotoxicosis.

Common side effects

At excessive doses there will be symptoms of thyrotoxicosis (eg sweating, palpitations, tremor, weight loss, heat intolerance).

Interactions

Enzyme-inducing drugs may accelerate the metabolism of thyroid hormones (see page 12).

Antithyroid drugs

Essential physiology

Hyperthyroidism is commonly caused by Graves' disease, which is mediated by thyroid-stimulating antibodies. Other common causes are toxic multinodular goitre and a toxic adenoma of the thyroid.

Thionamides

Mechanism of action

These antithyroid drugs act by interfering with the synthesis of thyroid hormone. They inhibit thyroid peroxidase-catalysed iodination of thyroglobulin in the thyroid. They also have some immunosuppressive effects.

Examples

- Carbimazole
- Propylthiouracil
- Methimazole.

Example prescription

CARBIMAZOLE 20 mg p.o o.d.

Standard dosages

Gradual dose titration

Carbimazole, the most commonly used thionamide, is given in high doses (40–60 mg daily) until the thyroid function tests are in the normal range. This usually takes 1–2 months. The dose is then reduced gradually to keep the thyroid function normal. Treatment is continued for a total of 18 months.

Block and replace

Alternatively, a combination of a full dose of carbimazole (40–60 mg) with levothyroxine (50–150 micrograms daily) can be given and continued for about 1 year. This is convenient, because less monitoring is needed. This regimen is unsuitable for use in pregnancy.

About 50% of patients suffer from relapse of hyperthyroidism. Treatment choices are then long-term low-dose antithyroid drugs, or radioactive iodine.

Indications

- Graves' disease
- Toxic multinodular goitre
- Toxic adenoma of the thyroid.

Absolute contraindication

Hypothyroidism.

Common side effects

- Rash and itch
- Alopecia
- Agranulocytosis is rare but life-threatening; all patients should be advised to report symptoms suggestive of infection, such as fever or sore throat; antithyroid drugs should be stopped if there is clinical or laboratory evidence of neutropenia
- Rarely, propylthiouracil can cause a lupus-like syndrome.

Significant interactions

None.

Radioactive iodine

Mechanism of action

Radioactive iodine (^{131}I) is treated as normal iodine by thyroid cells. Once taken up by active thyroid cells, radioactive iodine causes irreversible cell damage. This reduces function and, with time, some reduction in thyroid size can occur.

Standard dosages

The dose of radioactive iodine is chosen by the radiotherapist administering the drug. Dose depends on thyroid size and whether or not the aim is rapid induction if hypothyroidism.

Contra-indications

- Pregnancy
- Breast feeding
- Severe dysthyroid eye disease

Common side effects

- May cause a temporary increase in the symptoms of thyrotoxicosis (due to the release of stored hormone from the damaged gland)

Significant interactions

None

Other Drugs

Non-cardioselective β blockers are often used to control the symptoms of thyrotoxicosis until anti-thyroid drugs or radioactive iodine treatment takes effect. Propranolol, in a long acting preparation, is most commonly used (see page 52).

Corticosteroids

Corticosteroids are used in physiological replacement doses in deficiency states and in high doses when their anti-inflammatory properties are desirable. The general properties of glucocorticoids are described in this chapter, and reference to this section is made in other parts of the book that deal with conditions for which corticosteroids may be prescribed.

Corticosteroid replacement

Essential physiology

The adrenal cortex secretes both cortisol (hydrocortisone), which has glucocorticoid properties and weak mineralocorticoid effects, and aldosterone, which is a mineralocorticoid. The adrenal cortex is stimulated by adrenocorticotrophic hormone (ACTH) from the anterior pituitary. There is diurnal variation in cortisol secretion, with levels being higher in the morning and lower at night.

In primary adrenal insufficiency, both hydrocortisone and aldosterone need replacing. In hypopituitarism with secondary adrenal insufficiency however, a mineralocorticoid is not needed, because aldosterone production is regulated by the intact renin-angiotensin system.

Mechanism of action

Glucocorticoids are used in doses that give a serum level of cortisol as near normal as possible, with a normal diurnal variation in serum levels.

Examples

- Hydrocortisone
- Prednisolone
- Dexamethasone.

Example prescription

HYDROCORTISONE 15 mg p.o. mane, HYDROCORTISONE 5 mg p.o. at 6pm

Standard dosages

In the UK, hydrocortisone is most often used at a dose of 20–30 mg daily in divided doses, with the bigger dose given in the morning. In the USA, prednisolone 5 mg or 7.5 mg daily is widely used as adrenal replacement therapy.

Indications

- Primary adrenal insufficiency, commonly caused by Addison's disease
- Hypopituitarism
- After adrenalectomy.

Contraindication

Cushing's syndrome.

Common side effects

No significant side effects at physiological doses.

Significant interactions

See page 184.

Corticosteroids as anti-inflammatory therapy

Essential physiology

Corticosteroids are used in many conditions for their anti-inflammatory properties. It is their glucocorticoid activity that is anti-inflammatory, so those corticosteroids that have mainly mineralocorticoid activity, such as fludrocortisone, are not used as anti-inflammatories. Corticosteroids such as hydrocortisone, which have some mineralocorticoid activity, are used for emergency conditions, but not for long-term use because of the unwanted mineralocorticoid side effects.

Synthetic corticosteroids vary in their anti-inflammatory potency, and duration of action. The choice of glucocorticoid, dose and duration of treatment will depend on the severity and seriousness of the condition treated, its activity and the side effects of the glucocorticoid. Corticosteroids can be administered orally, intravenously, topically or by inhaler, depending on the condition to be treated and the specific medication chosen.

When long-term corticosteroids are used in chronic disease, the side effects can cause significant disability (eg osteoporosis, hyperglycaemia, myopathy, weight gain), so the maintenance dose should be kept as low as possible. If a patient is on corticosteroid treatment for more than three weeks, there will be suppression of adrenal function. Treatment must not be stopped suddenly or the patient will be at risk of acute adrenal insufficiency (see Addisonian crisis, p 192). Patients who are on or have recently stopped steroid therapy may need an increase in dose or a temporary re-introduction of costicosteroid treatment during acute illness or peri-operatively. Patients on long-term steroids should be advised to carry a Steroid Treatment Card.

Examples

For examples, see Table 7.1.

Corticosteroid	Glucocorticoid activity	Mineralocorticoid activity
Prednisolone 5 mg	++	0
Cortisone acetate 25 mg	++	+
Dexamethasone 750 micrograms	++	0
Hydrocortisone 20 mg	++	+

The doses listed are all equivalent to prednisolone 5 mg.
Physiological doses of steroids are equivalent to 7.5 mg prednisolone/day.

Table 7.1 Corticosteroids

Example prescription

PREDNISOLONE 60 mg p.o. o.d.

(This high dose might be used, for example, in the initial management of temporal arteritis.)

Indications

These are dealt with in appropriate sections in other chapters. Some examples are:

- Respiratory medicine: asthma, interstitial lung disease
- Gastroenterology: inflammatory bowel disease
- Rheumatology: inflammatory arthritis, vasculitis, temporal arteritis
- Palliative care: cerebral oedema.

Contraindication

Systemic infections.

Common side effects

- Hypertension
- Electrolyte imbalance
- Hyperglycaemia
- Osteoporosis
- Psychosis
- Proximal myopathy
- Cushing's syndrome.

Significant interactions

- Antagonism of antihypertensives
- Increased risk of bleeding when given with aspirin or NSAIDs
- Antagonism of oral hypoglycaemic drugs
- Antagonism of diuretics, and increased risk of hypokalaemia with thaizide diuretics.

Mineralocorticoids

Mineralocorticoids promote sodium and water resorption from the glomerular filtrate as it passes down the renal tubule. Lack of mineralocorticoid activity causes hyponatraemia, and intravascular hypovolaemia, which leads to hypotension, particularly after postural change.

Example

Fludrocortisone.

Example prescription

FLUDROCORTISONE 100 micrograms p.o. mane

Indications

- Adrenal insufficiency
- Postural hypotension in autonomic failure.

Absolute contraindications

- Hypertension
- Oedema
- Heart failure.

Common side effects

- Hypertension
- Electrolyte imbalance.

Significant interactions

Corticosteroid interactions, page 184

Bisphosphonates

Essential physiology

Bone is in a constant state of turnover, being continually formed and resorbed. Bone resorption is carried out by osteoclasts, which are derived from monocytes. Bone production is a function of osteoblasts, which are derived from fibroblast-like cells.

Bone mass starts to decrease after the age of 40 in both sexes, and occurs more rapidly in women after the menopause. Osteoporosis occurs when bone mass is critically reduced and there is loss of the structural integrity of the bone. Men have a higher bone mass than women, so osteoporosis-related fractures happen more often in women. Corticosteroids that promote gluconeogenesis from protein can cause osteoporosis in doses with glucocorticoid activity equivalent to > 7.5 mg prednisolone/day.

Mechanism of action

Bisphosphonates adsorb on to hydroxyapatite crystals in bone, and impair the ability of osteoclasts to adhere to the bone surface, thus inhibiting bone resorption.

Examples

- Pamidronate
- Risedronate
- Alendronate.

Standard dosages

Oral risedronate and alendronate can be given as a daily dose, or once weekly. Pamidronate is used mainly as an intravenous infusion for hypercalcaemia of malignancy.

Example prescription

RISEDRONATE 35 mg p.o. once weekly

Indications

- Osteoporosis
- Prophylaxis of corticosteroid-induced osteoporosis
- Paget's disease of bone
- Hypercalcaemia of malignancy.

Absolute contraindications

- Hypocalcaemia
- Pregnancy and breast-feeding.

Common side effects

- Nausea and vomiting
- Oesophageal ulceration and stricture: to minimise the chance of this, tablets should be taken without chewing, with fluid, while sitting or standing, at least 30 minutes before breakfast
- Rash
- Dizziness
- Headache.

Significant interactions

Absorption of bisphosphonates is reduced by antacids and calcium salts.

Drugs used in the treatment of breast cancer

Tamoxifen

Mechanism of action

Some types of breast cancer cells have oestrogen receptors. Binding of oestrogen to these receptors increases cell growth and promotes cancer development. Tamoxifen is an antagonist at such receptors and thus aims to limit the effects of oestrogen on breast cancer tissue.

Example prescription

TAMOXIFEN 20 mg p.o. o.d.

Indication

Oestrogen receptor positive breast cancer.

Contraindication

Pregnancy.

Common side effects

- Hot flushes
- Vaginal bleeding/discharge
- Risk of endometrial cancer
- Increased risk of thromboembolism.

Significant interaction

Increased anticoagulant effect of warfarin.

Anastrozole

Mechanism of action

Similar to tamoxifen, this drug is used for oestrogen receptor-positive breast cancer. It works by inhibiting the aromatase enzyme, which normally converts androgens to oestrogens. The circulating oestrogen level is thus reduced.

Example prescription

ANASTROZOLE 1 mg p.o. o.d.

Indication

Oestrogen receptor-positive breast cancer in patients who cannot take tamoxifen as a result of either the risk of thromboembolism or endometrial disease.

Contraindications

- Premenopausal women
- Pregnancy
- Breast-feeding
- Liver or renal impairment.

Common side effects

- Hot flushes
- Vaginal bleeding/dryness
- Gastrointestinal tract disturbance
- Bone fractures.

Significant interactions

None.

Trastuzumab (Herceptin®)

This is a monoclonal antibody which binds to human epidermal growth factor receptor-2 (HER2), which is found on certain breast cancer cells. By so doing, it blocks the action of human epidermal growth factor on the breast cancer cells, and thereby reduces cell division and growth. It is only suitable in selected cases, for tumours that overexpress HER2.

Oral contraceptive pills

Three preparations are in common use:

1. Monophasic combined oral contraceptives: these drugs contain a fixed amount of an oestrogen and a progestogen. The same dose of each hormone is therefore taken each day.

2. Biphasic and triphasic combined oral contraceptives: these drugs also contain an oestrogen and a progestogen, but the progestogen dose escalates throughout the month to mimic the natural hormonal cycle.

3. Progestogen-only contraceptives: these preparations contain no oestrogen components. They are often used when oestrogen-containing preparations are contraindicated.

Mechanism of action

Combined preparations act mainly to inhibit ovulation. They also have effects on the fallopian tubes and endometrial tissue, which reduces the chance of successful fertilisation and implantation. When given orally, progestogen-only contraceptives probably have little effect on ovulation, but have effects on cervical mucus and endometrial lining.

Examples

There are a great many preparations of oral contraceptive agents available. Alternative forms of contraception should always be discussed with the patient, to ensure that she can make an educated choice about contraception. Standard and low-strength preparations of combined pills are available and differ in the amount of oestrogen that they contain. The low-strength agents are generally chosen in patients at higher risk of cardiovascular disease.

Patches and implantable deposits of hormones are also available.

Indications

- Contraception
- Hypogonadism in females
- Hirsutism and acne

- Endometriosis
- Dysmenorrhoea.

Contraindications

Combined pills

- Patients with two or more risk factors for venous thromboembolism or arterial disease
- Certain types of migraine
- Pregnancy
- Systemic lupus erythematosus
- Breast cancer.

Progestogen-only pills

- Severe arterial disease
- Pregnancy
- Vaginal bleeding.

Common side effects

Combined pills

- Increased risk of venous thromboembolism with combined pills
- Nausea and/or vomiting
- Breast tenderness
- Skin pigmentation (cloasma).
- Fluid retention
- Hypertension
- Possible increased risk of breast cancer.

Progestogen-only pills

- Menstrual irregularity
- Nausea and/or vomiting
- Breast tenderness
- Mood changes
- Possible increased risk of breast cancer.

Significant interactions

- The contraceptive effect of oestrogens and progestogens is reduced by:
    - various antibiotics, antifungals and antiviral agents
    - various anticonvulsants
    - barbiturates
    - modafinil.
- Reduced anticoagulant effect of warfarin
- Progestogens increase plasma concentrations of ciclosporin.

Emergencies

Diabetic ketoacidosis

Diabetic ketoacidosis is characterised by a blood pH < 7.3, raised blood glucose, ketonuria, ketonaemia and dehydration. Patients often complain of nausea, vomiting, abdominal pain, and 'shortness of breath', which is actually hyperventilation or Kussmaul's breathing. In this hyperventilatory state, the patient is attempting to 'blow off' CO_2 which is produced by the buffering of excess H^+ by HCO_3^-. Ketoacidosis is caused by the build-up of excessive ketone bodies, produced by the metabolism of fat in the absence of sufficient insulin for aerobic metabolism. The principles of management of ketoacidosis are:

- Replacement of insulin, usually given as a continuous intravenous infusion of soluble insulin via an infusion pump
- Rehydration with intravenous saline
- Replacement of potassium chloride in the saline infusion to prevent hypokalaemia (insulin infusion + glucose causes a shift of K^+ intracellularly).

The dose of intravenous insulin is adjusted to maintain a blood sugar level between 5 mmol/l and 10 mmol/l. An insulin infusion is usually continued for 24–48 hours before a patient can return to their regular subcutaneous insulin.

Ketoacidosis is commonly precipitated by intercurrent illness, particularly when accompanied by vomiting or omission of insulin doses. The cause should be sought in all patients, and where remediable causes are found, the patient should be educated in an attempt to avoid recurrence of the ketoacidosis.

Hypoglycaemia

If the patient with hypoglycaemia is cooperative, oral glucose can be given by mouth; 20 g glucose can be given as four teaspoons of sugar or about 50 ml Lucozade®. This may have to be repeated again in about 10 minutes.

If the patient is unconscious, an injection of glucagon 1 mg can be given. Glucagon is a hormone produced by the a cells of the pancreatic islets, which mobilises glycogen from the liver. It can be given intravenously, intramuscularly or subcutaneously. Once the patient regains consciousness after being given glucagon, he or she should be given some oral carbohydrate.

In the hospital setting, an unconscious patient can be given intravenous dextrose for severe hypoglycaemia; 10 g glucose as 50 ml 20% glucose intravenous infusion can be given. The same amount of glucose could be given as 20 ml 50% glucose solution, but this concentration is very irritating to veins.

> **Never give 50% dextrose to children because of the risk of cerebral oedema.**

The cause of the hypoglycaemia (such as wrong dose of insulin or tablets, a missed snack or meal, unusual activity or alcohol excess) should be sought in all patients, and the patient should be adequately educated in an attempt to avoid recurrence of the hypoglycaemia.

Hypoglycaemia caused by oral hypoglycaemic drugs can persist for many hours because of the long half-life of these drugs, and patients usually need to be admitted to hospital for monitoring.

Thyrotoxic Crisis

Patients with life-threatening thyrotoxicosis (also called thyroid storm or thyroid crisis) have florid signs of thyrotoxicosis, fever, marked tachycardia, heart failure and disturbance of consciousness with delerium or coma. Nausea, vomiting and jaundice may also occur. The condition can occur in untreated patients, but it is often precipitated by an event such as thyroid surgery or radioactive iodine treatment or infection. The same drugs are used as in thyrotoxicosis but at high doses or by the intravenous route for rapid effect. Oral iodine can be given. This blocks the release of T 4 and T3 from the thyroid. A typical drug regimen would be:

- Propylthiouracil 200mg p.o. 6 hourly
- Metoprolol 5 mg i.v. or propranolol 80 mg 6 hourly until beta blockade achieved
- Iodine as Lugol's iodine p.o. (130 mg Iodine/ml)10 drops 8 hourly

Addisonian crisis

Acute adrenal insufficiency can be the presentation of Addison's disease or can occur in patients on adrenal replacement therapy who, through intercurrent illness or stress, have not taken their replacement therapy or have not absorbed it.

Patients are often shocked (low blood pressure and tachycardic), but symptoms can be non-specific, with anorexia, nausea, vomiting, abdominal pain, fatigue or confusion.

Adrenal crisis is treated by infusion of 0.9% sodium chloride, with hydrocortisone 100 mg i.v. 6- to 8-hourly. Large doses of fluid are often required (eg up to 6 litres in first 24 hours).

8
Fluids and electrolytes

8
Fluids and electrolytes

Although various preparations are available for use as intravenous fluids, the vast majority of patients can be managed using only three types of fluid:

1. Sodium chloride 0.9% (saline)

2. Dextrose 5%

3. Potassium chloride 0.3%.

> **In patients who have normal renal function and are capable of excreting excess fluid and electrolytes, precise fluid and electrolyte replacement is not essential, provided that the minimum daily requirement is given and excessive amounts are not infused.**

Sodium chloride 0.9%

This is the solution that results when 9 g sodium chloride (NaCl) is dissolved in 1 litre water. Each litre contains 150 mmol sodium ions (Na^+) and 150 mmol chloride ions (Cl^-). An adult with normal total body sodium and chloride levels requires 150 mmol of each of these ions daily, to maintain normal levels; 1 litre 0.9% saline given in 1 day will therefore provide the daily requirement of sodium and chloride as well as providing 1000 ml water. If a patient is deficient in sodium and/or chloride, then more than 1 litre will be required to replace the deficit (see below).

Dextrose 5%

This is an isotonic solution of 50 mg dextrose monohydrate in each millilitre of water. It is used to provide a source of water.

Intravenous fluid and electrolyte therapy

Box 8.1 Daily requirements of intravenous fluids

For adults with normal renal function the approximate daily requirements are:

Water   1.5–3.0 litres

Sodium   150 mmol

Chloride   150 mmol

Potassium 70 mmol

For individuals who are in normal fluid balance (neither dehydrated nor in a state of fluid overload), daily intravenous fluid and electrolyte balance will be maintained by giving the following fluids:

- 1 litre 0.9% saline + 20 mmol KCl over 8 hours
- 500 ml 5% dextrose + 20 mmol KCl over 8 hours
- 1 litre 5% dextrose + 30 mmol KCl over 8 hours.

If the person is dehydrated, an increased volume of 5% dextrose can be given. If the person is overhydrated, less 5% dextrose can be used.

Intravenous fluids in renal impairment

For patients with renal impairment, it is essential that the exact volume of fluid to be given is accurately determined.

Daily fluid requirement

A volume of fluid equivalent to 500 ml plus the total fluid output in the preceding 24 hours is required to keep fluid balance in steady state.

The extra 500 ml is required to replace the 'insensible' fluid volume that is lost each day in sweat, exhaled air, faeces, etc. Total output includes urinary volume plus any fluid volume lost in vomitus, surgical drains, blood loss and/or liquid faeces (diarrhoea).

If the patient has high Na^+ levels, the fluid given should be 5% dextrose. If Na^+ levels are normal, 0.9% saline can be used, but remember that most patients with renal impairment have elevated levels of potassium, so no additional KCl should be added to the fluids.

Management of hyponatraemia

Hyponatraemia is defined as a serum $Na^+ < 135$ mmol/l, and is the most common electrolyte abnormality found in hospitalised patients.

The mainstay of treatment is to identify and treat the underlying cause. If necessary, sodium can then be replaced if the patient is deficient, or a fluid restriction can be imposed.

Calculation of sodium deficiency

For normal adults, the total body water (in litres) is approximately 0.5 x body mass (kg).

$$\text{Total body water (l)} \approx 0.5 \times \text{body mass (kg)}$$

If a patient has a low serum Na^+, the Na^+ deficiency can be calculated as shown below.

$$Na^+ \text{ deficiency (mmol)} = \frac{(140 - N) \times M}{2}$$

where N is the patient's sodium level in millimoles per litre and M is the mass in kilograms.

Example

A 70-kg patient has a serum Na^+ of 130 mmol/l. The Na^+ deficiency is:

$$Na^+ \text{ deficiency} = \frac{(140 - 130) \times 70}{2} = 350 \text{ mmol}$$

As 1 litre of 0.9% saline contains 150 mmol Na^+, then:

$$350/150 = 2.33 \text{ litres } 0.9\% \text{ saline}$$

is required to replace the deficiency.

The daily fluid balance must be carefully monitored, and daily electrolytes should be measured to ensure that the sodium levels are returning to normal and potassium levels remain within the normal range.

Hypertonic saline (2.7% NaCl), which contains 462 mmol/l, should be used only after taking expert advice from senior medical staff, because sudden changes in Na^+ concentration can do more harm than good.

Management of hyperkalaemia

Degree of hyperkalaemia	Plasma K^+ level (mmol/l)
Mild	5.5–6.0
Moderate	6.1–6.9
Severe	≥ 7.0

Table 8.1 Degrees of hyperkalaemia

Don't forget

Severe hyperkalaemia is a medical emergency that requires urgent treatment.

1. Give 10 ml 10% calcium gluconate by slow intravenous infusion (over 2 minutes). This protects myocardial cells from the effect of hyperkalaemia; it has no effect on the level of potassium in the blood.

2. Give 50 ml 50% glucose infused over a period of 30 minutes.

3. Give 10 units soluble insulin intramuscularly 5–10 minutes after the start of the 50% glucose infusion.

4. Check K^+ level after 15–20 minutes. Repeat the dose of insulin and glucose, if the potassium level remains > 6 mmol/l.

5. Check blood glucose and serum K^+ after 30 minutes and repeat steps 2 + 3 if necessary.

6. Check blood sugar levels every 30 minutes for at least 6 hours and infuse 5% dextrose if blood glucose falls below normal (< 3.3 mmol/l).

7. Ion exchange resins can be given to help keep the K^+ level from rising again. These can be given by mouth or as an enema.

- 15 g calcium polystyrene sulphonate p.o. t.i.d., diluted in water

- 30 g in methylcellulose solution p.r. retained for 9 hours, followed by irrigation to remove resin from the colon.

If these measures fail peritoneal or haemodialysis are the only way to reduce and maintain the K^+ concentration within the normal range.

Management of hypokalaemia

Hypokalaemia most often results from diuretic drug therapy. It can also occur in patients receiving intravenous fluids without adequate potassium supplementation. This is a particular risk if the patient is losing excess K^+ by vomiting or diarrhoea or through surgical drains.

The average normal daily requirement of K^+ is 70 mmol, so patients receiving intravenous fluids should generally be given 20–40 mmol KCl in each litre of fluid. Patients with low levels of serum K^+ require the absolute deficiency to be calculated and then replaced. The calculation is similar to that for Na^+, shown earlier.

$$K^+ \text{ deficiency (mmol)} = \frac{(4 - K) \times M}{2}$$

where K is the patient's K^+ level in millimoles per litre and M is the mass in kilograms.

Example

A 80-kg patient has a serum K^+ of 2.8 mmol/l. The K^+ deficiency is:

$$K^+ \text{ deficiency} = \frac{(4 - 2.8) \times 80}{2} = 48 \text{ mmol.}$$

This patient therefore has an absolute K^+ deficiency of 48 mmol. This can be given as 48 ml 0.3% KCl solution, because this contains 1 mmol K^+/ml. To replace the deficiency and give the daily requirement without giving excess K^+ in 24 hours, 80 mmol KCl can be added to the intravenous fluids and slowly infused every 24 hours over a number of days (about 5 days) until the serum K^+ level is within the normal range. The serum K^+ concentration should be measured every 24 hours and carefully monitored.

Management of hypocalcaemia

Before treating hypocalcaemia it is important to determine the 'corrected' serum Ca^{2+} level, ie the level that is adjusted according to the patient's serum protein level.

> ### Calculating the corrected calcium level
>
> **For every 4 g/l that the albumin level is below 40 g/l add 0.1 mmol/l to the calcium level.**

Calcium should be given only if the corrected serum Ca^{2+} level is below the normal range, or to supplement the dietary calcium in patients who are taking bisphosphonates to prevent or treat osteoporosis.

Calcium can be given orally as one of many preparations. Examples include:

- Calcium gluconate 600 mg (1.35 mmol Ca^{2+})
- Calcium lactate 300 mg (1.0 mmol Ca^{2+})
- Calcium carbonate 500 mg (12.6 mmol Ca^{2+}).

α-colecalciferol is used to treat the hypocalcaemia associated with renal failure. This is because normal metabolism of vitamin D requires two hydroxylation steps: one in the liver to 25 hydroxy vitamin D, and the second in the kidney to 1,25 dihydroxy vitamin D. Patients with renal impairment are often unable to perform the second step, and they therefore require this to be given as an oral supplement.

If intravenous replacement is deemed necessary, 10% calcium gluconate can be given. This contains 220 micromoles per millilitre (μmol/ml); 10 ml are given by very slow (ie not less than 2 minutes) intravenous injection or diluted in 250 or 500 ml 0.9% saline or 5% dextrose and infused over a period of 2–4 hours.

Management of hypercalcaemia

As for hypocalcaemia, it is important to ensure that the 'corrected' calcium level is determined (ie adjusted for any abnormality in serum protein), and also that any high level is checked by a repeat serum calcium analysis performed on an uncuffed blood sample (prolonged use of a tourniquet can cause a false elevation of the serum Ca^{2+} level).

For severe hypercalcaemia the following treatments are used:

- Intravenous infusion of 5% dextrose and 0.9% saline: 4–6 litres in the first 24 hours, followed by 3–4 litres daily for several days. This will rehydrate the patient because hypercalcaemia causes polyuria and may also be associated with vomiting.

- Disodium pamidronate: 15–60 mg in 0.9% saline or 5% dextrose, infused over a period of 4–6 hours once per day and repeated for up to 4 days.

- Calcitonin: 200 units intravenously. This drug has a very short action and is used only to rapidly reduce an extremely high calcium level until rehydration and bisphosphonates have time to work.

- Prednisolone: 30–60 mg p.o. This is effective in reducing the hypercalcaemia associated with sarcoidosis, multiple myeloma and excessive vitamin D.

Management of hypomagnesaemia

A serum magnesium level < 0.7 mmol/l requires correction.

This can be done by giving 50 mmol magnesium chloride in 1 litre 5% dextrose or 0.9% saline infused over 12–24 hours. The infusion can be repeated if the serum Mg^{2+} concentration remains low on repeat testing.

Management of hypermagnesaemia

Hypermagnesaemia describes a serum Mg^{2+} concentration of > 2.0 mmol/l.

Treatment is by infusing 10 ml 10% calcium gluconate in 100 ml 5% dextrose over 20 minutes. Then 10 units of soluble insulin are added to 50 ml 50% glucose and should also be given by slow intravenous injection (over a period of 5–10 minutes). This treatment reduces not only the serum Mg^{2+} but also the serum K^+, and therefore both electrolytes should be carefully monitored. For very severe cases of hypermagnesaemia, haemodialysis may be required.

9
Musculoskeletal system

Analgesics
Disease modifying drugs for rheumatoid arthritis
Drugs used to treat gout

9
Musculoskeletal system

Analgesics

Essential physiology

Pain is one of the most common symptoms of disease and often one of the earliest manifestations of an underlying disorder. It is essential that patients can be prescribed adequate pain relief (analgesia).

The sensation of pain arises by activation of peripheral sensory receptors; the axons from these are mainly in the spinothalamic tract and, to a much lesser extent, in the dorsal columns of the spinal cord, both terminating at the thalamus.

Cutaneous pain differs considerably from visceral or deep pain. Cutaneous pain can usually be specifically localised to the point of stimulation whereas deep or visceral pain cannot be localised accurately.

Pain relief can be achieved in a number of ways:

- Blocking the peripheral sensory receptors, eg local anaesthetic agents
- Blocking the spinal cord axon pathways, eg spinal block anaesthesia
- Blocking pain sensation at the level of the thalamus ± affecting pain sensation by acting on the limbic system.

Most drug therapies used aim to block the perception of pain at the thalamus (ie central pain receptors). These agents are described in this chapter.

Non-opioid analgesics

These drugs are much less likely to cause central nervous system (CNS) depression or addiction than opiate drugs. Their ability to relieve pain varies from drug to drug and a spectrum of analgesic properties is a useful concept to consider when deciding which pain-relieving drugs should be prescribed (see below).

Pain score	Suitable analgesic
1	Aspirin
2	Paracetamol
3	NSAIDs
4	Codeine
5	Dihydrocodeine
6	Tramadol
7	Pethidine
8	Pentazocine
9	Morphine
10	Diamorphine

NSAIDs, non-steroidal anti-inflammatory drugs.

Table 9.1 Matching the analgesic to the pain; IO = worst pain

Aspirin (acetylsalicylic acid)

Mechanism of action

Aspirin has a number of properties apart from its action as an analgesic. It also acts as an antipyretic to reduce fever and inhibits platelet aggregation, so reducing the risk of intravascular clot formation. Its analgesic properties are weak. Its mechanism of action is described on page 236.

Example prescription

ASPIRIN 300–600 mg p.o. q.i.d.

Indication

Mild to moderate pain.

Contraindications

- Patients under 16 years of age (risk of Reye's syndrome)
- Breast-feeding
- Peptic ulceration.

Common side effects

- Gastric irritation (less with enteric-coated preparations)
- Peptic ulceration

- Bronchospasm and/or anaphylaxis in aspirin-sensitive individuals
- Increased bleeding time.

Significant interactions

Aspirin is metabolised in the liver to its active metabolite salicylic acid, which is bound to the protein albumin in the circulation. The drug can therefore affect the pharmacokinetics of other protein-bound drugs, eg warfarin. There is an increased risk of bleeding when aspirin is combined with other antiplatelet agents or anticoagulants.

Paracetamol

Mechanism of action

This drug can be used to reduce fever. It has no direct anti-inflammatory activity. Paracetamol acts both at peripheral sensory neurones and at the level of the thalamus to block pain perception.

Example prescription

PARACETAMOL 1 g 4- to 6-hourly p.r.n., maximum 4 g/day

Indication

Mild to moderate pain.

Contraindications

None.

Common side effects

- Skin rashes
- Hepatic impairment (especially in overdose in patients with liver disease).

Significant interactions

None.

Non-steroidal anti-inflammatory drugs (NSAIDs)

Mechanism of action

These drugs act by inhibiting the action of the cyclo-oxygenase COX-1 and COX-2 enzymes, which are involved in arachidonic acid metabolism (Figure 9.1).

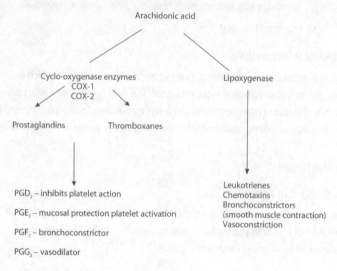

Figure 9.1 Products of arachidonic acid metabolism.

COX-1 is an enzyme produced in small amounts by normal cells and is responsible for maintaining the integrity of tissues, eg it is responsible for inhibiting platelet aggregation, maintaining blood flow and preventing mucosal cell damage.

COX-2, on the other hand, is upregulated in cells by the action of the cytokines during inflammatory reactions. Cells such as vascular endothelial cells, macrophages and synovial fibroblasts, as well as neutrophils and lymphocytes, produce increased quantities of COX-2, which results in the production of thromboxanes that cause platelet aggregation, vasoconstriction and other proinflammatory and pain-producing mediators (including excessive prostaglandin PGE_2). Different NSAIDs have different relative effects on the two enzymes. In general, selective COX-2 inhibitors are associated with fewer side effects such as gastric irritation or ulceration and are less likely to affect platelet aggregation.

Until recently, COX-2 inhibitors were believed to be much safer than non-selective COX inhibitors. However, there is now significant evidence that some selective COX-2 inhibitors are associated with increased incidence of myocardial infarction (MI) and cerebrovascular events in patients with a personal or family history of these conditions. They should therefore not be prescribed in patients who have these conditions or other risk factors associated with ischaemic heart disease or strokes.

Additional actions of NSAIDs include:

- Anti-inflammatory: reduce chemotaxins at the site of inflammation
- Antipyretic: inhibit prostaglandin activity in the hypothalamus
- Antithrombotic: inhibit platelet aggregation resulting from reduced thromboxane A_2 synthesis.

Examples

- Naproxen
- Indometacin
- Diclofenac
- Ibuprofen
- Meloxicam
- Celecoxib.

Example prescription

IBUPROFEN 400 mg p.o. t.i.d.

Indication

Moderate pain.

Contraindications

NSAIDs should be avoided in:

- Elderly patients
- Patients with NSAID hypersensitivity
- Pregnancy and breast-feeding
- Impaired renal function
- Peptic ulceration
- Asthma.

Selective inhibitors of COX-2 should not be prescribed for:

- Patients with a personal history of ischaemic heart disease or stroke
- Patients with a family history of ischaemic heart disease or stroke
- Patients with risk factors for cardiovascular disease.

Common side effects

- Dyspepsia
- Gastric erosions/ulceration
- Renal impairment
- Hypersensitivity reactions – bronchospasm/anaphylaxis
- Bleeding
- Dizziness, vertigo
- Fluid retention
- COX-2-selective NSAIDs increase the risk of MI and/or stroke in at-risk patients.

Significant interactions

Most NSAIDs are protein bound and will therefore compete for binding sites with other drugs such as warfarin.

> ### Note
>
> NSAIDs can cause severe bronchospasm, angioedema and/or anaphylactoid reactions in about 2% of the population. These individuals are said to be aspirin- and NSAID-hypersensitive. If they take these drugs, the cyclo-oxygenase pathway is completely blocked and all arachidonic acid metabolism occurs via the lipoxygenase pathway. The production of high levels of leukotrienes causes severe and prolonged bronchospasm, and the activation of cytokines from inflammatory cells can cause widespread mast cell degranulation.

Opioid (narcotic) analgesics

Mechanism of action

Not only do these drugs relieve pain but they also either induce sleep or suppress the level of consciousness. They are extremely powerful pain relievers but have addictive properties, especially when used at high dosage or over a period of time. They can cause both physical and psychological dependence.

They act by binding to receptors on the presynaptic membrane of the pain-carrying neurones and to receptors in the thalamus and limbic system in the brain. Binding to these receptors has several effects:

- Analgesia
- Respiratory centre suppression
- Sedation
- Nausea
- Miosis (pupillary constriction)
- Feeling of wellbeing
- Physical dependence.

All of the opiates apart from diamorphine can be given as oral medication. For severe pain, intravenous medication achieves higher plasma levels. Most have a short half-life (about 4–6 hours).

Examples

- Morphine
- Diamorphine
- Codeine
- Dihydrocodeine
- Pentazocine
- Pethidine
- Tramadol.

Example prescriptions

TRAMADOL 100 mg p.o. 4- to 6-hourly p.r.n., maximum 400 mg/day

DIAMORPHINE 2.5–5 mg s.c. or i.m. or i.v. 4-hourly p.r.n.

MORPHINE 5–10 mg s.c. or i.m. or i.v. 4-hourly p.r.n.

Indications

These drugs are best used for moderate to severe pain and for visceral pain.

Contraindications

- Respiratory depression
- Alcohol intoxication
- Paralytic ileus
- Head injury, raised intracranial pressure.

Common side effects

- Respiratory depression
- Nausea ± vomiting
- Constipation
- Itch
- Physical dependence
- Withdrawal symptoms.

Don't forget

Always prescribe an antiemetic alongside an opiate analgesic, and also consider prescribing a laxative.

Significant interactions

None.

Box 9.1 Analgesia for common medical conditions

General principles

- Treat the underlying cause of the pain if possible.

- Use an analgesic dosage regimen that prevents pain – it is easier to prevent pain than to achieve pain relief once it is established.

- Use adequate doses to achieve pain relief, but not excessive dosages or potency.

- Potent intravenous drugs should be diluted and given slowly.

- All potent analgesics (opiates) can cause respiratory depression.

- Patients with renal and/or hepatic disease and elderly patients are at increased risk of drug overdose and unwanted effects.

- Do not use strong analgesia if it might mask the symptoms of peritonitis.

- Opiates are more likely to cause respiratory depression in patients with liver and/or renal impairment or in patients with respiratory failure and/or chronic lung disease.

Examples of suitable analgesia for a variety of medical conditions are listed below:

Myocardial infarction
MORPHINE SULPHATE 5–10 mg i.v. 4-hourly p.r.n.

Plus antiemetic, eg CYCLIZINE 50 mg i.v. 8-hourly p.r.n.

or

DIAMORPHINE 2.5–5 mg i.v. 4-hourly p.r.n.

Plus antiemetic, eg CYCLIZINE 50 mg i.v. 8-hourly p.r.n.

Headache
Mild: PARACETAMOL 1 g p.o. 4–6 hourly p.r.n. Maximum 4 g/day.

Moderate: CO-CODAMOL 30/500 mg p.o. one to two tablets 4- to 6-hourly p.r.n. Maximum eight tablets per day (contains paracetamol 500 mg and codeine phosphate 30 mg per tablet)

Severe: DIHYDROCODEINE 30 mg p.o. 4- to 6-hourly p.r.n. or TRAMADOL 50-100 mg p.o. 4- to 6-hourly. Maximum 400 mg/day

Musculoskeletal pain
PARACETAMOL 1 g p.o. 4- to 6-hourly p.r.n. Maximum 4 g/day

Box 9.1 Analgesia for common medical conditions *(continued)*

or

CO-CODAMOL 8/500 mg p.o. one to two tablets 4- to 6-hourly p.r.n. Maximum eight tablets/day (contains paracetamol 500 mg and codeine phosphate 8 mg per tablet)

or

IBUPROFEN 400 mg p.o. 8-hourly p.r.n.

Postoperative pain
Check ward/hospital policy – most surgical units/anaesthetic departments have an analgesic policy that should be consulted and used.

Colic
Acute biliary colic: strong analgesic together with antispasmodic

Acute renal colic: PETHIDINE 50–100 mg i.v. 6-HOURLY p.r.n.

Plus HYOSCINE BUTYLBROMIDE 20 mg p.o. q.i.d.

or

PROPANTHELINE BROMIDE 15 mg p.o. t.i.d.

Neuropathic pain
Trigeminal neuralgia: CARBAMAZEPINE 100–200 mg p.o. b.d.

Postherpetic pain: simple analgesia + AMITRIPTYLINE 50–75 mg o.d. p.o. ± GABAPENTIN (300 mg o.d. on day 1, 300 mg b.d. on day 2, then 300 mg t.i.d. with a gradual reduction in dose when the patient is pain free)

Noctural leg muscle cramps
QUININE SULPHATE 200–300 mg p.o. nocte

Pain relief for patients with cancer
Pain relief is an important part of palliative care, which includes many other aspects, such as psychological, social and spiritual care. Advice should be sought from a palliative care team and/or hospice to plan adequate pain relief tailored to the needs of individual patients and their families.

As a general principle, the number of drugs used should be as few as possible and if oral medication cannot be used parenteral medication may be required, sometimes as subcutaneous infusions delivered by syringe drivers or patient-controlled administration.

Disease-modifying drugs for rheumatoid arthritis

Essential physiology

To understand the rationale for using drugs in this condition, it is helpful to have some understanding of the pathophysiology of the inflammatory process involved.

Rheumatoid arthritis is a multisystem, non-organ-specific autoimmune disorder in which circulating immune complexes become deposited in small blood vessels and subsequently activate an inflammatory reaction. The immune complexes are made up of autoantibody (rheumatoid factor) combined with a self-antigen (the patient's own immunoglobulin IgG).

Although immune complex deposition can occur in blood vessels of any tissue, they have a predisposition for vessels of the synovial membrane of joints. The major clinical manifestations are therefore an inflammatory arthritis that eventually leads to a deforming arthritis.

When immune complexes attach to receptors on the endothelial cells of synovial vessels they activate complement. This in turn causes the production of complement degradation products, which act as chemotaxins, attracting inflammatory cells including neutrophils, lymphocytes and monocytes/macrophages.

Neutrophils migrate out of the vessels into the synovial tissue and the joint space, where they release proteolytic enzymes that damage cartilage, synovium and supporting tissues (ligaments and tendons). Lymphocytes and macrophages release cytokines, including tumour necrosis factor (TNF), which stimulate proliferation of cells of the synovium. The synovium then grows over and invades cartilage and nearby bone. Some cytokines are also responsible for new blood vessel formation (angioneogenesis) and fibroblast proliferation within the synovial membranes.

The following drugs are used to control the *symptoms* of the disease:

- Paracetamol
- Aspirin
- NSAIDs.

Disease-modifying antirheumatic drugs (DMARDs) are used to reduce the action of inflammatory cells and have little or no direct analgesic effect. They are used together with analgesic agents. These are a number of drugs used. They are started early in the course of rheumatoid arthritis, to prevent joint damage. They may be considered if pain and inflammation continue after 2–3 months on an NSAID.

Antimalarials

Mechanism of action

The exact mode of action of this group is poorly understood but it is thought that these drugs inhibit the release of chemotaxins and inhibit lymphocyte transformation and cytokine release. They may also inhibit the action of antigen-presenting cells (macrophages)

Examples

- Chloroquine
- Hydroxychloroquine.

Example prescriptions

CHLOROQUINE 150 mg p.o. o.d.

HYDROXYCHLOROQUINE 100–200 mg p.o. b.d.

Indications, contraindications, common side effects and significant interactions

See page 282.

Penicillamine

Mechanism of action

Penicillamine is thought to act in a number of ways in inhibiting the inflammatory process. It may stabilise the cell membranes of inflammatory cells and their lysosomal membranes. It is also thought to reduce the production of immunoglobulins, and may therefore reduce the production of rheumatoid factor and antibody production to new antigens expressed during the process of cartilage and synovial damage.

The drug is a chelating agent, so it can also be used in the treatment of iron overdose and Wilson's disease (an inherited disorder associated with excessive copper in the body).

Example prescription

PENICILLAMINE 125–250 mg p.o. o.d.

Indications

- Rheumatoid arthritis
- Iron poisoning
- Wilson's disease.

Contraindication

Systemic lupus erythematosus (SLE).

Common side effects

These are common and affect about one in three patients who are given this drug:

- Nausea and vomiting
- Oral ulceration
- Fever
- Bone marrow suppression
- Skin rash
- Proteinuria (may lead to nephrotic syndrome)
- Loss of taste
- Haematuria
- Stevens–Johnson syndrome.

Significant interaction

As a result of its chelating properties, its absorption is reduced in patients taking oral iron therapies and vice versa.

Immunosuppressives

Immunosuppressive drugs act by suppressing both cell-mediated and antibody-mediated immune reactions. They inhibit antibody production, cytokine release and the activity of the antigen-presenting cells.

Antimetabolites

Methotrexate
See page 243.

Example prescription

> METHOTREXATE 7.5 mg p.o. once per week

Azathioprine
See page 241.

Example prescription

> AZATHIOPRINE 25–50 mg p.o. b.d.

Alkylating agents

Cyclophosphamide
See page 242.

Example prescription

> CYCLOPHOSPHAMIDE 25–50 mg p.o. o.d. or b.d.

Immunomodulating drugs

Ciclosporin
See page 240.

Example prescription

> CICLOSPORIN 1.25 mg/kg p.o. b.d.

Entanercept

Mechanism of action

This drug is produced by recombinant technology. It consists of two TNF receptors (TNF$_R$) fused to the Fc portion of human IgG. It is used to inhibit immunological reactions that are triggered by TNF. Free TNF (and/or TNF-β) is mopped up by the TNF$_R$ and so TNF's effect is inhibited. The drug is used to treat active rheumatoid arthritis and inflammatory bowel disease (IBD).

The drug must be given by injection. It has a long half-life (5–7 days), so subcutaneous injection of 25 mg twice each week is sufficient to achieve a therapeutic level.

Example prescription

ENTANERCEPT 25 mg s.c. twice per week

Indications

- Rheumatoid arthritis
- IBD
- Severe psoriasis.

Contraindications

- Active infection
- Pregnancy
- Breast-feeding.

Common side effects

- Increased risk of infection, including tuberculosis (TB)
- Potential increased risk of malignancy
- Risk of exacerbation of demyelinating disease
- Renal impairment
- Myositis
- Local reaction at injection sites
- Lymphadenopathy.

Significant interaction

This drug should not be given with live vaccines.

Infliximab

Mechanism of action

This is a monoclonal antibody that consists of mouse anti-human TNF linked to human IgG antibody. When infused, it binds to human TNF and inhibits the inflammatory responses triggered by this cytokine. Similar to entanercept, it is used to treat active rheumatoid arthritis and IBD as well as other immunological disorders including vasculitis.

It has no effect on TNF-β, because the mouse monoclonal antibody is specific for the α form.

This drug must be given by intravenous infusion. It has a half-life of about 21 days. Therefore, once a plasma level has been achieved by giving 3 mg/kg body weight slowly by intravenous infusion, and repeated after 2 and 6 weeks, infusions given once every 2 months are sufficient to achieve the desired anti-inflammatory effect.

Example prescription

> INFLIXIMAB 2 mg/kg intravenous infusion repeated at 2 weeks and 6 weeks, then every 8 weeks

Indications

- Rheumatoid arthritis
- IBD.

Contraindications

- Active infection
- Pregnancy
- Breast-feeding.

Common side effects

- Increased risk of infection, including TB
- Increased risk of malignancy
- Hypersensitivity reactions – angioedema and urticaria
- Fever
- Skin rashes
- Anaphylaxis

- Hepatitis
- Interstitial pneumonitis/pulmonary fibrosis
- Seizures
- Demyelination.

Significant interaction

This drug should not be given with live vaccines.

Other DMARDs eg gold and sulphasalazine are also used under specialist supervision.

Drugs used to treat gout

Essential physiology

Gout is a type of inflammatory arthritis characterised by raised levels of uric acid in the blood with the formation of uric acid crystals in synovial fluid. Uric acid is produced when the body metabolises purines. Xanthine oxidase is the enzyme responsible for the last stage in purine metabolism.

Drugs used for the acute attack

NSAIDs

See page 203.

Example prescription

DICLOFENAC 50 mg p.o. 8-hourly p.r.n.

Colchicine

Mechanism of action

Colchicine interferes with normal cell mitosis, by inhibiting cellular microtubular assembly. It thereby reduces leukocyte activation and interferes with the function of some proinflammatory mediators.

Example prescription

COLCHICINE 1 mg p.o., followed by 500 micrograms 2- to 3-hourly p.r.n. until pain free or until vomiting or diarrhoea occurs; maximum dose 6 mg

Indications

- Acute gout
- Prophylaxis of acute gout when starting allopurinol.

Contraindication

Pregnancy.

Common side effects

- Nausea and vomiting
- Diarrhoea.

Significant interaction

There is increased risk of toxicity when colchicine is prescribed with ciclosporin.

Prednisolone (see page 182)

Uncommonly, this drug can be given if NSAIDs and colchicine cannot be used. One must be sure that the joint inflammation is not caused by infection before starting this therapy. Steroid joint injections may also be used in acute gout.

Drugs used to prevent gout

Allopurinol

Mechanism of action

Allopurinol is an inhibitor of xanthine oxidase, so it reduces the synthesis of uric acid in the body; it is given prophylactically in patients prone to attacks of gout.

Example prescription

ALLOPURINOL 200 mg p.o. o.d.

Indications

- Prophylaxis of gout
- Prophylaxis of renal calculi
- Concomitant prescription with certain types of chemotherapy to prevent hyperuricaemia associated with cell destruction.

Contraindications (see box)

> **Allopurinol should never be started during an acute flare of gout. The patient should wait around 1 month before starting this agent.**
>
> **If, however, an acute attack of gout occurs when a patient is already on allopurinol, the drug should be continued and the acute flare treated as detailed above.**

> **Starting allopurinol**
>
> **Commencement of allopurinol may trigger an acute attack of gout. Colchicine or an NSAID should be prescribed alongside allopurinol, and should continue for 1 month after the hyperuricaemia has been corrected.**

Common side effects

- Rash
- Gastrointestinal tract disturbance.

Significant interaction

Co-prescription of allopurinol with azathioprine causes increased toxicity.

10
Haematology and immunology

Haematology and
Immunology

10
Haematology and immunology

Haematinics

Haematinics are substances that are required for the manufacture of erythrocytes (red blood cells).

Iron

Mechanism of action

Iron is best absorbed from the upper small bowel in the ferrous (Fe^{2+}) state. It is transported across intestinal cells and into the plasma. Iron in the plasma is carried to developing red cells in the bone marrow by a protein called transferrin.

The normal adult diet contains about 5 mg iron per 1000 calories of food. Of this, 10% gets absorbed. Most dietary iron is in the ferric (Fe^{3+}) form. Iron absorption is increased in iron-deficiency states and if iron therapy is given together with vitamin C (ascorbic acid), which aids the conversion of ferric to ferrous iron. The daily iron requirement for men is 1 mg/day and for premenopausal women it is 2 mg/day.

For patients with iron-deficiency anaemia, therapy should be continued until the haemoglobin level remains stable within the normal range and then for a further 3 months. This period of time is necessary to allow the total body iron stores to be replenished.

Examples

Oral iron

- Ferrous sulphate
- Ferrous fumarate
- Ferrous gluconate.

Parenteral iron

This form of therapy is used only for patients who cannot tolerate oral iron preparations – because of unwanted or intractable side effects – or for patients with malabsorption states. These preparations can be given either by deep intramuscular injection or by slow intravenous infusion.

- Iron dextran: a complex of ferric hydroxide and dextran containing 5% iron
- Iron sucrose: a complex of ferric hydroxide and sucrose containing 2% iron.

Example prescription

FERROUS FUMARATE 210 mg p.o. t.i.d.

Calculation of parenteral iron dosage

This is done according to the body weight of the patient and the iron deficit, which is determined from either a table or a graph that accompanies the product literature.

Indication

Iron-deficiency anaemia.

Contraindications

Parenteral iron is contraindicated in people with:

- Allergic disorders
- Active rheumatoid arthritis
- Liver disease
- Infection.

Common side effects

Oral iron

- Nausea
- Dyspepsia
- Altered bowel habit (diarrhoea or constipation)
- Darkening the colour of the stools.

Intramuscular iron

- Staining of injection site
- Pain at injection site
- Metallic taste
- Arthralgia.

Intravenous iron

- Flushing
- Headache
- Bronchospasm
- Urticaria
- Myalgia
- Arthralgia
- Nausea/vomiting
- Fever
- Anaphylaxis.

Administration of intravenous iron

Because of the risks of anaphylaxis during the infusion, facilities for resuscitation should always be available. The risk of a serious reaction is increased in patients with allergic diseases (eg asthma, eczema), inflammatory disorders (eg active rheumatoid arthritis, systemic lupus erythematosus [SLE]) and hepatic or renal impairment. In addition, patients who have been given parenteral iron should not be given an oral preparation for at least 5 days.

Significant interactions

Absorption of oral iron salts is adversely affected by the use of antacids.

Vitamin B_{12} (hydroxycobalamin)

Mechanism of action

Absorption of dietary vitamin B_{12} requires the formation of a complex with a glycoprotein known as intrinsic factor, produced by the parietal cells of the stomach. The vitamin B_{12}–intrinsic factor complex binds to receptors of the terminal ileum where vitamin B_{12} absorption takes place over a period of about 8 hours.

The main dietary source of vitamin B_{12} is red meat (especially offal such as liver) and dairy products (milk, cheese and eggs), and to a much lesser extent vegetables.

As most deficiency states are the result of problems with absorption, treatment is given by intramuscular injection in the form of hydroxycobalamin.

Example prescription

To replace deficiency in uncomplicated pernicious anaemia:

> HYDROXOCOBALAMIN 1 mg i.m. three times per week for 2 weeks, then
>
> HYDROXOCOBALAMIN 1 mg i.m. once every 3 months

Indication

Vitamin B_{12} deficiency.

Contraindications

None.

Common side effects

- Nausea
- Hypersensitivity reactions (uncommon).

Significant interactions

None.

Folic acid

Mechanism of action

Folic acid is mainly absorbed in the duodenum and jejunum. It is obtained as folates from fresh leaf vegetables and red meat or offal (especially liver). Folate is necessary during pregnancy and is used prophylactically to protect the fetus from neural tube defects such as spina bifida.

Example prescription

FOLIC ACID 5 mg p.o. o.d.

This dose should be taken for 4 months in folate deficiency states. In pregnancy, the 5-mg dose is generally used when there is high risk of a neural tube defect (eg parent or previous child affected). When the risk is lower, 400 micrograms/day can be used. Folic acid should ideally be taken before conception, and continued until week 12 of pregnancy.

Indications

- Folic acid deficiency
- Prophylaxis of neural tube defects in pregnancy.

Contraindications

Don't forget

Never prescribe folic acid on its own for patients who are likely to be vitamin B_{12} deficient. This practice can precipitate subacute combined degeneration of the spinal cord.

Common side effects

None.

Significant interactions

None.

Erythropoietin

Mechanism of action

This hormone is normally released from the juxtaglomerular cells of the kidney in response to hypoxia, and stimulates red blood cell production in the bone marrow. It is used to treat the normochromic/normocytic anaemia associated with chronic renal failure. Human erythropoietin is produced for therapeutic use by recombinant DNA technology.

Example prescription

EPOETIN BETA 2000 units s.c. three times per week for 4 weeks

Erythropoietin is given at a dose of 50 units/kg body weight one to three times per week until the haemoglobin and red blood cell counts are within the desired range, but at a rate not exceeding 2 g/dl haemoglobin per month. Adequate iron stores are essential and therefore this treatment is often used together with oral iron therapy.

> Erythropoietin should not be given by subcutaneous injection to patients with chronic renal failure, but can be used subcutaneously for other conditions as described below.

Indications

- Anaemia associated with chronic renal failure
- Anaemia resulting from cancer chemotherapy
- To increase yield of autologous blood in bone marrow pre-donation programmes
- To treat the anaemia associated with AIDS or HIV infection.

Contraindication

Severe hypertension.

Common side effects

- Fever
- Myalgia
- Hypertension
- Thrombosis of arteriovenous shunts in renal dialysis patients.

Significant interactions

None.

Anticoagulants

Any drug that inhibits the formation of a blood clot (thrombus) is, by definition, an anticoagulant. Unlike fibrinolytic drugs (see page 72), anticoagulants have little, if any, effect on a thrombus once it has formed. They are therefore mainly used as prophylactic agents with the aim of preventing blood clot formation. They are used in a variety of clinical settings as shown in Box 10.1.

Box 10.1 Indications for prophylactic anticoagulation

- Atrial fibrillation

- History of deep venous thrombosis

- History of pulmonary embolism

- Carotid artery stenosis

- Transient ischaemic attacks

- Myocardial infarction

- Unstable angina

- Patients who are immobilised, eg fracture patients

- Preoperatively and postoperatively

- Antiphospholipid antibody syndrome

- Thrombophilia or other hypercoagulable states, including major trauma or malignancy

- Prosthetic heart valves

In patients with deep vein thrombosis (DVT) and/or pulmonary embolism (PE), anticoagulants prevent extension of thrombus and therefore reduce the risk of small portions of poorly organised new clot breaking off and causing further problems. They also prevent further new thrombus formation. In the setting of a PE, anticoagulants not only prevent further embolism but also reduce the area of pulmonary infarction that develops (Figure 10.1).

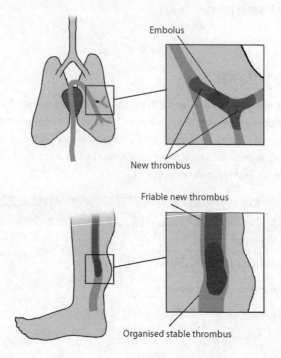

Figure 10.1 Anticoagulants aim to reduce thrombus extension as shown.

There are two main anticoagulants used in clinical practice: heparin and warfarin.

Heparin

Mechanism of action

This is a mucopolysaccharide (glycosaminoglycan) that binds to and activates a circulating natural anticoagulant protein called antithrombin. The heparin–antithrombin complex inhibits the action of a number of activated clotting factors in the coagulation cascade (IXa, Xa, XIa and XIIa). It also binds directly to thrombin and inhibits its ability to convert fibrinogen to fibrin.

Heparin must be given by injection because it is inactivated in the gastrointestinal tract. Onset of action is almost immediate once it enters the blood.

Heparin can be used as an unfractionated molecule (molecular mass 20–30 kDa), or as low-molecular-mass molecules (molecular masses around 7 kDa).

Unfractionated heparin has a very short half-life, which depends on the dosage and the route of administration. Low-molecular-weight heparins (LMWHs) have a much longer duration of action and half-life because they do not bind to plasma proteins or to endothelial cells. LMWH is the drug of choice in pregnant women who require anticoagulation.

Heparin flushes are used to maintain the patency of venous and/or arterial cannulae. They prevent backwash of blood, thereby reducing the risk of thrombus formation and blockage. Box 10.2 explains how to monitor heparin.

Box 10.2 Monitoring anticoagulation with heparin

For unfractionated heparin, the degree of anticoagulation is monitored by measuring the activated partial thromboplastin time (APTT) with the aim of therapy to keep the APTT between 1.5 and 2 times normal.

As LMWHs have a much more predictable effect, provided that the correct dosage is given, routine monitoring is not required.

Examples

- Unfractionated heparin
- Enoxaparin (low molecular weight).

Example prescription

Unfractionated heparin

Given by intravenous infusion or injection every 4–6 hours. For doses, see Box 10.4.

LMWH

Given by subcutaneous injection once or twice daily. For doses, see Box 10.4.

Heparin flushes

HEPARIN SODIUM 10 units/ml in 0.9% SALINE – 5 ml i.v. every 4–6 hours

Indications

See Box 10.4.

Contraindications

- Bleeding disorders
- Recent severe bleeding
- Severe hypertension
- Severe liver disease.

Common side effects

- Haemorrhage
- Osteoporosis – usually only after prolonged use
- Heparin-induced thrombocytopenia
- Hyperkalaemia
- Urticaria and angioedema.

Significant interactions

Reversal of heparin: 1 mg protamine sulphate neutralises 80–100 units heparin. Protamine sulphate is given by very slow intravenous injection (over a period of 10–15 minutes). As a result of the short half-life of heparin, the amount of protamine sulphate needed decreases with time after heparin has been given.

Warfarin

Mechanism of action

Warfarin is an orally administered drug; it is the most commonly used anticoagulant for long-term therapy of thromboembolic disorders. It acts by inhibiting a reductase enzyme in the liver that is necessary in the conversion of vitamin K to its active form. If the active vitamin K is not present, the hepatic synthesis of vitamin K-dependent clotting factors (II [prothrombin], VII, IX and X) is reduced. The onset of anticoagulation is delayed until the quantities of preformed clotting factors have been depleted.

Warfarin is well absorbed when given by mouth and binds to plasma proteins in the circulation. It is metabolised in the liver by the cytochrome P450 enzyme system and has a long half-life (about 24 hours). As the plasma concentration does not correlate with its anticoagulant activity, plasma levels cannot be used to assess its control of coagulation. Rather, a test known as the 'international normalised ratio' (INR) is used. The INR is based on the prolongation of the prothrombin time. The degree of prolongation is compared with that of a sample of control plasma, and the dose of warfarin is adjusted in an attempt to achieve the desired INR. The target therapeutic ranges for the INR differ according to the condition being treated, as shown in Table 10.1. As a general rule, an INR of about 3.0 is ideal for most conditions.

Condition	Target INR
Prophylaxis of deep venous thrombosis	2.0–2.5
Treatment of deep venous thrombosis and pulmonary embolism	2.0–3.0
Treatment of atrial fibrillation	2.0–3.0
Prophylaxis in patients with prosthetic heart valves	3.0–4.0
Recurrent deep venous thrombosis or pulmonary embolism in patients on warfarin with therapeutic INR	3.0–4.0

Table 10.1 Target international normalised ratio (INR) ranges for a variety of conditions

Example prescription

WARFARIN as per INR p.o o.d.

Starting warfarin therapy

There is a lag phase between starting warfarin therapy and the onset of anticoagulant action. This results from the fact that all the preformed vitamin K-dependent clotting factors have to be depleted before warfarin's full anticoagulant activity is apparent. The lag phase varies between individuals, depending on a variety of factors, including body mass, liver cell function and rate of utilisation of clotting factors. To achieve adequate anticoagulation reasonably quickly, it is necessary to initiate warfarin therapy using dose titration. A recommended regimen is shown in Table 10.2.

Day	Warfarin dose (mg)	INR check required?
1	9	No
2	6	No
3	6	Yes
4	3	Yes
5	3–6 depending on day 4 INR	Yes
6	0–6 depending on day 5 INR	Yes
Subsequently	1–9 depending on INR	Yes

Table 10.2 Recommended regimen for warfarin

Indications

See Box 10.4.

Contraindications

- Recent severe bleeding
- Severe hypertension
- Severe liver disease.

Common side effects

- Haemorrhage (see Box 10.3)
- Birth defects – warfarin should not be given to women who are pregnant or breast-feeding
- Alopecia
- Skin rashes
- Liver impairment.

Box 10. 3 Bleeding and warfarin

Bleeding is the main unwanted effect of warfarin, and can occur if the patient takes excessive amounts of the drug, or drugs or alcohol which can affect the plasma concentration. The risk of haemorrhage is reduced if the INR is monitored regularly and the dose of warfarin adjusted to keep the INR within the desired therapeutic range. If the INR exceeds the range, omission of the drug and/or reducing the dose often prevents any bleeding tendency.

Management of major bleeding

- Stop warfarin

- Give vitamin K (PHYTOMENADIONE) 5 mg by slow intravenous injection

- Give either

    - fresh frozen plasma (FFP; 15 ml/kg body weight) or

    - prothrombin complex concentrate (50 units/kg body weight) as a source of factors II, VII, IX and X

Management of minor bleeding or an INR > 8.0

- Stop warfarin

- Measure INR regularly, ie once or twice per day

- Restart warfarin at a reduced dose when INR < 5.0

- If the patient has other risk factors for bleeding or if bleeding continues, give 5 mg vitamin K by slow intravenous injection

Management of an INR > 6.0

- Stop warfarin

- Regular INR measurements (once per day)

- Restart warfarin at a reduced dose when INR < 5.0 at lower dosage

Management of unexpected bleeding with INR within therapeutic range

- Stop warfarin

- Investigate for other cause of bleeding

Significant interactions

A number of drugs can affect the anticoagulant effect of warfarin by a variety of mechanisms:

- Displacing warfarin from protein-binding sites: this increases the amount of free drug in the circulation and therefore increases the anticoagulant effect, eg oral contraceptive pill, non-steroidal anti-inflammatory drugs, steroids.

- Inducing cytochrome P450 enzyme systems (see page 12): this reduces the anticoagulant effect, eg anticonvulsant drugs.

- Inhibiting cytochrome P450 enzyme systems (see page 12): this increases the anticoagulant effect, eg cimetidine, amiodarone.

- Reducing production of vitamin K-dependent clotting factors: this increases the anticoagulant effect, eg various antibiotics.

When prescribing a drug for a patient who is taking warfarin, it is essential to check for possible drug interactions and in particular what potential effect the drug may have on the INR. See Box 10.4 for treatment of important thromboembolic conditions.

Box 10.4 Treatment of important thromboembolic conditions

Deep venous thrombosis

Prophylaxis

ENOXAPARIN 20–40 mg s.c. o.d. In preoperative patients, give first dose 2 hours before surgery.

Treatment

- ENOXAPARIN 1.5 mg/kg s.c. o.d. for 5 days minimum and until adequate oral anticoagulation is established

- Start warfarin therapy day on day 1 using dosage titration (see Box 10.2) to achieve a stable INR of 2.0–3.0

For the first DVT, continue oral anticoagulation for 3 months.

For the second DVT, continue oral anticoagulation for 6 months.

For the third or subsequent DVT, investigate for an underlying cause and give warfarin for life.

Box 10.4 Treatment of important thromboembolic conditions (continued)

Pulmonary embolism (PE)

- ENOXAPARIN 1.5 mg/kg s.c. o.d. until adequate oral anticoagulation achieved
- Start warfarin on day 1 using dosage titration (see Box 10.2) to achieve a stable INR of 2.0–3.0

For the first episode of PE, continue treatment for 6 months.

For the second or subsequent PE, investigate for an underlying cause and give warfarin for life.

Unstable angina

Unfractionated heparin; loading dose: 5000 units i.v., followed by a continuous infusion of 15–25 units/kg body weight per hour.

Acute peripheral arterial occlusion

Enoxaparin 1 mg/kg s.c. b.d.

As for unstable angina.

Hospitalised patient post-myocardial infarction with moderate to severe cardiac failure

ENOXAPARIN 40 mg s.c. o.d. for 6 days or until ambulant.

Antiplatelet drugs

There are a number of drugs that are used to prevent platelet activation or aggregation and so reduce the risk of platelet emboli and/or the initiation of intravascular coagulation. These drugs are used for prophylaxis in a variety of medical conditions as shown in Box 10.5.

Box 10.5 Uses for antiplatelet drugs

- Transient ischaemic attacks

- Carotid artery stenosis

- Ischaemic heart disease (angina pectoris)

- Secondary prevention after myocardial infarction

- After coronary artery bypass grafting or angioplasty ± stent insertion

- Thrombophilia

- Anti-phospholipid antibody syndrome

- Peripheral vascular insufficiency

Aspirin

Mechanism of action

Aspirin is a cyclo-oxygenase (COX) inhibitor that reduces the production of thromboxane A_2 by platelets. This reduces the ability of platelets to aggregate. Aspirin is capable of achieving this inhibition of platelet aggregation even at very low dosage, which prevents activation of intravascular coagulation without impairing normal blood clotting in response to trauma. At the low dosage used, the drug has little if any analgesic or anti-inflammatory properties, and the risk of unwanted effects is extremely low.

Example prescription

ASPIRIN 75 mg p.o. o.d.

Indications

For antiplatelet indications, see Box 10.5.

Contraindications, common side effects and significant interactions

See page 202.

Dipyridamole

Mechanism of action

This drug inhibits the enzyme phosphodiesterase, thereby increasing the level of cAMP within platelets. This results in reduced platelet aggregation because of a reduction in the expression of glycoprotein receptors. These receptors (GPIIb and GPIIIa) normally cross-link fibrinogen during blood clot formation, and also cause platelets to adhere to each other.

Example prescription

DIPYRIDAMOLE 200 mg p.o. t.i.d.

Indications

See Box 10.6.

Contraindications

None.

Common side effects

- Headache and may exacerbate migraine
- Dizziness
- Myalgia
- Hypotension ± tachycardia
- Worsening of angina pectoris
- Skin rashes, including urticaria.

Significant interactions

Dipyridamole enhances the effects of adenosine (see page 80). Adenosine should not be given to patients on this drug. There is an increased risk of bleeding if administered with warfarin.

Clopidogrel

Mechanism of action

This drug irreversibly binds to receptors on the platelet surface that normally bind to adenosine diphosphate (ADP). As a result, calcium mobilisation within platelets is reduced, resulting in reduced expression of the glycoprotein GPIIb and GPIIIa receptors. Platelet adhesion and platelet function are therefore impaired.

The drug has a half-life of 8–10 hours, but, because the binding to platelets is irreversible, a once-daily dosage regimen is sufficient to achieve a therapeutic effect.

Example prescription

CLOPIDOGREL 75 mg p.o. o.d.

Indications

See Box 10.6.

Contraindications

- Bleeding
- Breast-feeding.

Common side effects

- Dyspepsia
- Diarrhoea
- Haemorrhage
- Flatulence
- Dizziness
- Skin rashes
- Pancreatitits
- Hepatitis.

Significant interactions

There is an increased risk of bleeding if administered with warfarin.

Box 10.6 summarises the treatment of common conditions that need antiplatelet therapy.

Box 10.6 Treatment of common conditions requiring antiplatelet therapy

Transient ischaemic attacks and carotid artery stenosis

ASPIRIN 75 mg o.d. and DIPYRIDAMOLE 200 mg t.i.d. for 2 years. Then reduce to one drug thereafter.

If the patient cannot take aspirin then give DIPYRIDAMOLE 200 mg t.i.d. for 2 years. Then reduce to 100 mg t.i.d.

Ischaemic heart disease/secondary prevention of MI

ASPIRIN 75 mg o.d. ± CLOPIDOGREL 75 mg o.d.

If the patient cannot take aspirin then give CLOPIDOGREL 75 mg o.d. or DIPYRIDAMOLE 100 mg t.i.d.

Thrombophilia

ASPIRIN 75 mg o.d. ± CLOPIDOGREL 75 mg o.d.

Anti-phospholipid syndrome

ASPIRIN 75 mg o.d. or CLOPIDOGREL 75 mg o.d. or, if antibody level is very high or thromboembolism occurs, warfarin therapy is required.

Peripheral vascular insufficiency

ASPIRIN 75 mg o.d. ± CLOPIDOGREL 75 mg o.d.

Immunosuppressive drugs

Any drug that causes bone marrow suppression or inhibits cell proliferation will impair immune responses. There are a wide variety of drugs that suppress the immune system; however, only a small group of drugs is commonly used to treat medical conditions in which the immunological response is responsible for the disease (Box 10.7).

Box 10.7 Common medical conditions treated with immunosuppressive drugs

- Systemic lupus erythematosus (SLE)

- Vasculitis, eg polyarteritis nodosa, Wegener's granulomatosis

- Rheumatoid arthritis

- Inflammatory bowel disease

- Autoimmune liver disease

Limited knowledge of these drugs is required at undergraduate level, so a brief overview only is given here. These drugs should be prescribed only by specialists.

Ciclosporin

Mechanism of action

Ciclosporin is a peptide product of a fungus. It binds to cell surface receptors (calcineurin receptors) on helper T lymphocytes and inhibits calcineurin phosphatase, an intracellular enzyme. This enzyme is normally required for interleukin-2 (IL-2) production when the cells are stimulated by antigen. Failure to generate IL-2 results in downregulation of both cell-mediated and antibody-mediated reactions.

The drug is used mainly to prevent transplant tissue and/or organ rejection but is also useful in the treatment of autoimmune disorders. Once-daily dosing therapy is usually sufficient; however, plasma trough levels should be monitored to reduce the risk of toxicity.

Common side effects

- Renal impairment (common) – monitoring of renal function is essential
- Hypertension
- Hypertrichosis (excessive hair growth)
- Headache
- Liver cell damage
- Gum hypertrophy
- Anorexia, nausea ± vomiting
- Burning paraesthesiae of hands and feet
- Skin rashes
- Gout
- Pancreatitis
- Convulsions.

Azathioprine

Mechanism of action

This drug is an antiproliferative immunosuppressive that is often used, either alone or together with steroid therapy, to prevent organ transplant rejection and treat autoimmune disorders. It acts by interfering with the biosynthesis of purine and therefore DNA replication. Azathioprine is converted to the active metabolite 6-mercaptopurine, which competes with purines for incorporation into the DNA molecule.

Common side effects

- Bone marrow suppression
- Nausea ± vomiting
- Hair loss.

Significant interactions

The co-prescription of allopurinol can cause increased toxicity.

Mycophenolate

Mechanism of action

This is also an antiproliferative drug. It is metabolised to mycophenolic acid. The drug acts by inhibiting the enzyme inosine monophosphate dehydrogenase, thereby blocking the conversion of inosine monophosphate to xanthine monophosphate. Cells that are depleted of xanthine cannot synthesise DNA. This is particularly important for DNA synthesis in lymphocytes.

Significant side effects

- Bone marrow suppression
- Increased risk of infection
- Nausea ± vomiting
- Diarrhoea
- Hepatitis
- Pancreatitis.

Cyclophosphamide

Mechanism of action

This is an alkylating agent that is used extensively in cancer chemotherapy. It acts by damaging DNA, thereby interfering with cell replication. Cyclophosphamide contains reactive sites that covalently bind to DNA and other proteins, and inhibit DNA and RNA synthesis. After absorption, the drug is metabolised into two active products, acrolein and phosphoramide, which are excreted by the kidneys and are very irritant to the bladder surface.

Significant side effects

- Haemorrhagic cystitis
- Bone marrow suppression
- Azoospermia in males
- Anorexia, nausea and/or vomiting
- Hair loss at high dosage.

Methotrexate

Mechanism of action

This drug is an antimetabolite that acts by inhibiting the enzyme dihydrofolate reductase, thus interfering with the normal metabolic pathway for folic acid. Folic acid is essential for DNA recombination, and methotrexate therefore inhibits the normal cell cycle. The drug is used for cancer chemotherapy (especially for leukaemia and lymphoma), but can also be used at lower dosage for inflammatory conditions, especially rheumatoid arthritis or psoriasis.

Some drug remains bound to the dihydrofolate reductase enzyme for prolonged periods of time. A once-weekly dosage regimen is therefore usually sufficient to give the desired degree of immunosuppression. Folic acid is commonly co-prescribed with methotrexate to minimise the risks of folic acid deficiency.

Significant side effects

- Bone marrow suppression
- Liver cell damage
- Pleural effusion
- Pneumonitis.

Prednisolone

This drug is extensively used as an immunosuppressive agent in a wide variety of immunologically mediated conditions. Details can be found on page 182.

Drugs for the treatment of allergy

Essential physiology

Allergic disorders are forms of type 1 hypersensitivity reactions, which are mediated by antigen-specific immunoglobulin E (IgE) binding to mast cells. Some individuals have a tendency to produce IgE in response to innocuous substances in their environment and are described as 'atopic'. Atopic people tend to have asthma, eczema, allergic rhinitis or allergic conjunctivitis. The IgE that they produce (to a variety of substances) binds to mast cells throughout their body and, on subsequent exposure, antigen cross-linking of two IgE molecules causes the mast cell membrane to rupture with the release of preformed mediators, including histamine. With the rupture of the mast cell membrane, one of its constituents (arachidonic acid) is metabolised, leading to the production of a variety of prostaglandins and leukotrienes (Figure 10.2).

These chemical mediators are responsible for the late-phase reaction of the allergic response, comprising inflammatory changes, smooth muscle contraction and oedema. There are a number of sites where drug therapy can be used to treat allergic disease, as shown in Figure 10.3.

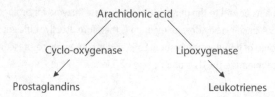

Figure 10.2 Metabolism of arachidonic acid.

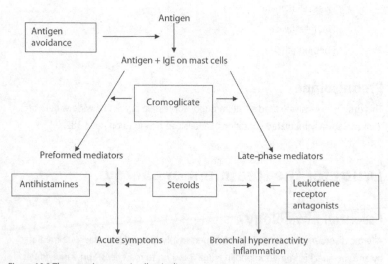

Figure 10.3 Therapeutic targets in allergic disease.

Drug reactions are a common cause of secondary urticaria and/or angioedema. Although these conditions can occur with a wide variety of drugs, they are recognised as common side effects of several agents (Box 10.8).

> ## Box 10.8 Drugs that cause urticaria and/or angioedema
>
> - Penicillin in penicillin-allergic individuals
> - Angiotension-converting enzyme (ACE) inhibitors
> - Angiotension-II receptor antagonists
> - Non-steroidal anti-inflammatory drugs (NSAIDs)
> - Codeine
> - Opiate analgesics

Mast cell stabilisers

Mechanism of action

All of these drugs are derived from cromoglicate compounds. Although it is generally thought that they stabilise the mast cell membrane, the exact mechanism by which they prevent mast cell membrane rupture is unknown. They prevent the release of preformed mediators and the subsequent production of the late-phase reactants.

Examples

- Sodium cromoglicate
- Nedocromil sodium.

Example prescription

SODIUM CROMOGLICATE 10 mg inhaled q.i.d.

Indications

Prophylaxis of:

- Asthma
- Allergic rhinitis
- Allergic conjunctivitis.

Contraindications

None.

Common side effects

- Inhalation of dry powder can cause bronchospasm, cough and throat irritation
- Headache
- Nausea and/or vomiting
- Abdominal pains
- Nasal irritation (nasal spray only)
- Transient burning/stinging of eyes (eye drops only).

Significant interactions

None.

Antihistamines

Mechanism of action

The drugs used here are selective type 1 histamine (H_1)-receptor blocking drugs that usually act as competitive inhibitors. They act by blocking the histamine receptors on vascular cells, smooth muscle fibres and nerve endings, and thus the vascular and neurological effects (vasodilatation, increased vascular permeability, smooth muscle contraction and itch) are suppressed.

Most of the newer, non-sedating antihistamines have a long half-life which means that they give satisfactory plasma levels on a once-a-day dosage regime.

Examples

Non-sedating

- Desloratadine
- Fexofenadine
- Levocetirizine
- Terfenadine.

Sedating

- Chlorphenamine
- Hydroxyzine.

Example prescription

DESLORATADINE 5 mg p.o. o.d.

Patients are often well controlled with a non-sedating preparation, but for acute attacks may require the addition of chlorphenamine. Occasionally, a combination of two antihistamines is required to keep symptoms controlled.

For severe cases the use of a non-sedating preparation taken in the morning and a sedating preparation at night is often useful.

> ### Don't forget
>
> Patients taking sedating antihistamines should be advised not to drink alcohol, drive or work with machinery.

Indications

Relief from allergic reactions, including urticaria.

Absolute contraindication

Some are contraindicated in porphyria.

Relative contraindications

- Urinary retention
- Prostatic hypertrophy
- Hepatic impairment
- Renal impairment.

Common side effects

- Sedation (with sedating preparations)
- Dry mouth
- Ventricular arrhythmias (with terfenadine)
- Potentiation of alcohol effects.

All of the side effects associated with this class of drug are much more common with the older, sedating antihistamines.

Significant interactions

There is a significant risk of ventricular arrhythmias when terfenadine is co-prescribed with many other drugs.

Bronchodilators

See page 91.

Leukotriene receptor antagonists

Mechanism of action

This class of drug blocks the effects of leukotrienes. They therefore reduce or prevent smooth muscle contraction and the chemotaxins that result in the inflammatory processes around ruptured mast cells. They are effective in asthma (both allergic and exercise-induced) when used alone or together with inhaled corticosteroids.

Examples

- Montelukast
- Zafirlukast.

Example prescription

MONTELUKAST 10 mg p.o. nocte

Indication

Prophylaxis of asthma.

Contraindications

- Pregnancy
- Breast-feeding
- Churg–Strauss syndrome.

Common side effects

- Gastrointestinal tract upset
- Dry mouth
- Thirst
- Hypersensitivity reactions.

Significant interactions

None.

Steroids

As a result of the adverse effects associated with steroid treatment, prednisolone should be used only for patients with severe allergic attacks that cannot be controlled with maximal antihistamine therapy. If they are required, the minimal effective dose needed to control symptoms should be used. Details are given on page 182.

Adrenaline (epinephrine)

Adrenaline is used to treat severe life-threatening angioedema and anaphylactic shock. See page 250 for further details. Box 10.9 details the treatment of hereditary angioedema.

Box 10.9 Hereditary angioedema

This condition is a rare autosomal dominantly inherited disorder in which there is an absolute deficiency of C1-esterase inhibitor in the circulation. Episodes of severe angioedema can be triggered by infection or physical trauma, including surgical procedures. Acute life-threatening laryngeal oedema can occur. Treatment can be with one of the following.

C1-esterase inhibitor

Acute attacks of angioedema can be treated with either fresh frozen plasma FFP or a purified derivative of fresh plasma – C1-esterase inhibitor concentrate. In addition, these preparations can be used prophylactically to treat patients before any surgical procedure, including dental extraction, that could potentially precipitate a severe attack. A dose of 1000–1500 IU of concentrate is often sufficient to abort an acute attack and 500–1000 IU as prophylaxis 1–2 hours before and after surgery.

Danazol

This drug has androgenic activity and the property of increasing the amount of C1-esterase inhibitor in the circulation. It can be used in a dose of 200 mg two or three times a day to prevent acute attacks of angioedema. In women, it can cause some virilisation, however.

Tranexamic acid

This antifibrinolytic drug, which inhibits fibrin dissolution, also has the property of increasing C1 esterase inhibitor levels. It can be used in a dose of 1–1.5 g two to three times daily to reduce the frequency and/or severity of acute attacks of angioedema. The major contraindication and side effect is thromboembolism.

Management of anaphylactic shock

Anaphylactic shock is an acute medical emergency that occurs as a result of widespread mast cell degranulation. It is usually triggered by an antigen entering the bloodstream of patients who have been sensitised to that specific antigen. The management is as follows:

- Secure the airway and provide 100% oxygen.

- Give adrenaline (epinephrine) 0.5 ml of 1:1000 dilution (1 mg/ml) intramuscularly, repeated after 5 minutes if no initial response.

- Give chlorphenamine 8 mg i.v.

- Give hydrocortisone 250 mg i.v.

- Give bronchodilators by nebuliser if bronchospasm is a manifestation.

- Provide an intravenous fluid infusion to maintain a systolic blood pressure of > 90 mmHg.

Patients who are at risk of acute anaphylaxis should have access to an antihistamine (eg chlorphenamine 4 mg) and a self-administration adrenaline (epinephrine) syringe that delivers a dose of 300 micrograms. They should be advised that at the first signs of an acute reaction occurring they should take 8 mg chlorphenamine by mouth. If symptoms persist or they develop shortness of breath or upper airway obstruction, they should urgently seek medical attention, preferably at a hospital accident and emergency department. If they have extreme difficulty breathing or feel faint they should self-administer a dose of adrenaline using the self-administration syringe.

11
Antimicrobial agents

Antibiotics
Antiviral drugs
Antifungal drugs
Antiparasitic drugs

11
Antimicrobial agents

These drugs are used to treat disease caused by micro-organisms, including bacteria (antibiotics), viruses (antiviral drugs), fungi (antifungals), protozoal organisms and helminths (antiparasitic drugs).

Antibiotics

Antibiotics can be divided into those that inhibit bacterial division (bacteriostatic agents), and those that kill the organisms (bactericidal agents). They may also be considered in terms of their mode of action, which can involve the following:

- Disruption of or damage to bacterial cell walls by either
    - inhibition of cell wall synthesis or
    - damage to cell walls by increasing permeability
- Alteration or inhibition of bacterial protein synthesis
- Blocking of metabolic pathways
- Prevention of DNA or RNA replication.

Within each group, individual drugs can also be classified as either broad spectrum or narrow spectrum, depending on whether they damage or destroy a wide or limited range of bacterial organisms.

Inhibitors of cell wall synthesis

These drugs contain a chemical structure known as the β-lactam ring which is responsible for preventing bacterial cell wall synthesis (Figure 11.1). The β-lactam antibiotics include the most commonly used antibiotics – penicillins and cephalosporins.

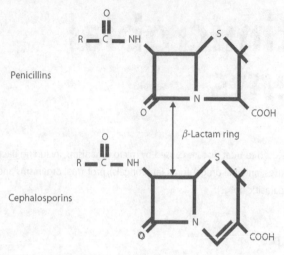

Figure 11.1 The chemical structure of penicillins and cephalosporins.

Pencillins

Mechanism of action

The β lactams inhibit the synthesis of the peptidoglycan layer of bacterial cell walls that surround certain bacteria. The bacteria rupture as a result of defective cell walls. Some organisms can, however, synthesise an enzyme (β lactamase) that can break down the β lactam ring and thus render the organisms resistant to this group of antibiotics. It is possible to overcome this resistance by combining the antibiotic with a β lactamase inhibitor (for example, clavulanic acid).

Examples

- Benzylpenicillin is quickly broken down in the stomach and therefore is best given by intramuscular or intravenous injection.

- Phenoxymethylpenicillin is more stable in an acid environment and can be given by mouth.

- Flucloxacillin, amoxicillin and ampicillin are well absorbed from the gastrointestinal tract. They can also be given parenterally.

- Co-amoxiclav consists of amoxicillin combined with clavulanic acid, a β-lactamase inhibitor. This drug is therefore active against resistant strains of *Staphylococcus aureus*, *Escherichia coli* and *Haemophilus influenzae* as well as many of the *Bacteroides* and *Klebsiella* species.

Example prescriptions

BENZYLPENICILLIN (PENICILLIN G) 1.2 g i.v. q.i.d.

PHENOXYMETHYLPENICILLIN (PENICILLIN V) 500 mg p.o. q.i.d.

CO-AMOXICLAV 625 mg p.o. t.i.d.

Contraindication

Penicillin hypersensitivity.

Common side effects

- Hypersensitivity reactions: erythematous or urticarial rashes, angioedema and/or anaphylaxis, fever or the Stevens–Johnson syndrome
- Seizures (if high serum levels are reached, for example in patients with renal failure)
- Diarrhoea.

Significant interactions

Probenecid is a uricosuric agent that reduces the excretion of penicillin. It is sometimes employed to ensure that high plasma levels of penicillin are achieved.

Cephalosporins

Mechanism of action

These drugs contain a β-lactam ring linked to a dihydrothiazine ring. This makes this class of drug resistant to the action of β-lactamase enzymes.

Some of these drugs (the early or first-generation cephalosporins) are well absorbed when given orally, whereas the drugs developed later (third- and fourth-generation drugs) must be given by intramuscular or intravenous routes.

Examples

- Cefalexin
- Cefuroxime
- Cefotaxime.

Example prescription

CEFOTAXIME 1 g i.v. b.d.

Contraindications

Probenecid reduces the excretion of these drugs. They can increase the anticoagulant action of warfarin.

Common side effects

- Nausea and vomiting
- Skin rashes
- Hypersensitivity reactions (more common in patients with penicillin allergy)
- Diarrhoea.

Agents that damage bacterial cell walls by increasing permeability

Polymyxins

Mechanism of action

These compounds bind to phospholipid molecules on bacterial cell walls and alter their permeability. This results in cell death by lysis. These drugs are active against Gram-negative organisms only. They are used mainly in the treatment of pseudomonas infections.

Pharmacokinetics

This class of drug is not absorbed when given by mouth and so for systemic infection it is given by intravenous infusion. It is excreted by the kidneys and has a half-life of about 12 hours.

The fact that it is not absorbed from the gut means that it can be used orally for sterilisation of the bowel.

Example

Colistin is the only polymyxin in current use.

Example prescription

COLISTIN 1 million units i.v. infusion t.i.d.

Contraindications

- Myasthenia gravis
- Pregnancy
- Breast-feeding.

Common side effects

- Impaired renal function
- Dizziness
- Convulsions
- Perioral paraesthesiae
- Confusion
- Skin rashes.

Significant interactions

There is an increased risk of toxicity when prescribed with ciclosporin or platinum cytotoxic agents. Colistin reduces the effects of drugs used to treat myasthenia gravis.

Vancomycin

Mechanism of action

This is a high molecular mass glycopeptide that inhibits bacterial cell wall synthesis by disrupting the formation of the normal peptidoglycan constituents. It is bactericidal to Gram-positive bacteria, especially staphylococci. It is also used to treat pseudomembanous colitis, caused by *Clostridium difficile* colonisation of the colon. This condition occurs when normal bowel commensals are destroyed by other antibiotic therapy. For systemic infections, this drug must be given by injection because it is poorly absorbed by mouth. However, for pseudomembanous colitis, it is best given by the oral route because high concentrations are achieved in the colon.

Example prescriptions

VANCOMYCIN 500 mg i.v. infusion q.i.d. (for example, for staphylococcal septicaemia)

VANCOMYCIN 250 mg p.o. q.i.d. (for pseudomembanous colitis)

Common side effects

- Thrombophlebitis
- Skin rashes (including generalised erythema)
- Ototoxicity
- Bone marrow suppression.

Significant interactions

There is an increased risk of nephrotoxicity when co-prescribed with ciclosporin and an increased risk of ototoxicity when co-prescribed with loop diuretics.

Drugs that alter bacterial protein synthesis

Macrolides

Mechanism of action

These drugs bind to bacterial ribosomes and interfere with protein synthesis. Their action is mainly bacteriostatic, and they are well absorbed when given by mouth, although erythromycin preparations must be given as enteric-coated tablets or an ester pro-drug, because the acidity of the stomach causes it to break down. Clarithromycin remains stable in an acid pH. This class of drug is often chosen in place of a penicillin if the patient is allergic to penicillin.

Examples

- Erythromycin
- Clarithromycin
- Azithromycin.

Example prescription

ERYTHROMYCIN 500 mg p.o. q.i.d.

CLARITHROMYCIN 250 mg p.o. b.d.

Contraindication

Caution must be exercised when used in patients with liver impairment.

Common side effects

- Nausea and/or vomiting (less so for clarithromycin)

- Diarrhoea
- Skin rashes
- Cholestatic jaundice
- Cardiac arrhythmias.

Significant interactions

The most common interaction relates to enhancing the anticoagulant effect of warfarin. Macrolides have multiple interactions; see Appendix 1 in the BNF for further details.

Aminoglycosides

Mechanism of action

These drugs also bind to a subunit of bacterial ribosomes, inhibiting protein synthesis and resulting in misreading of the genetic code. They must be given by injection because they are poorly absorbed from the gastrointestinal tract. Excretion is via the kidneys and they have short half-lives. As a result of potential serious neurotoxicity, particularly to the eighth cranial nerve, peak and trough concentrations must be carefully monitored.

Examples

- Gentamicin
- Amikacin
- Tobramycin.

Example prescription

GENTAMICIN 80 mg i.v. t.i.d.

Contraindication

Myasthenia gravis.

Common side effects

- Nephrotoxicity
- Ototoxicity.

Significant interactions

There is an increased risk of nephrotoxicity when co-prescribed with ciclosporin and an increased risk of ototoxicity when co-prescribed with loop diuretics.

Lincosamides

Mechanism of action

These drugs inhibit protein synthesis within bacteria in a similar way to the macrolides. They have excellent tissue penetration and are often used for staphylococcal bone infection (osteomyelitis).

Example

Clindamycin is the only lincosamide in current use.

Example prescription

Clindamycin 300 mg p.o. q.i.d.

Contraindication

Diarrhoea.

Common side effects

- Nausea and vomiting
- Pseudomembranous colitis
- Derangement of liver function
- Skin rashes.

Significant interactions

None.

Sodium fusidate (fusidic acid)

Mechanism of action

This narrow-spectrum antibiotic is a steroid that inhibits bacterial protein synthesis by preventing transfer RNA (tRNA) from binding to ribosomes. It has good penetration into tissues, including synovial fluid. Fusidic acid is often prescribed in addition to another antibiotic because resistance would be expected if it was used alone.

Example prescription

SODIUM FUSIDATE 500 mg p.o. t.i.d.

Contraindications

None.

Common side effects

- Nausea and/or vomiting
- Jaundice and derangement of liver function.

Significant interactions

None.

Tetracyclines

Mechanism of action

This group of antibiotics binds to a subunit of bacterial ribosomes and blocks protein synthesis. They are bacteriostatic rather than bactericidal. They have good tissue permeability except into cerebrospinal fluid. Tetracyclines are concentrated in the liver, excreted in bile and partially reabsorbed from the small intestine. Bile concentrations of the drug may therefore be three to five times higher than the serum concentration.

Examples

- Tetracycline
- Oxytetracycline
- Doxycycline.

Example prescription

DOXYCYCLINE 200 mg p.o. stat, then 100 mg p.o. o.d.

Contraindications

- Children (aged < 12 years)
- Pregnancy
- Breast-feeding.

Most are contraindicated in renal failure.

Common side effects

- Nausea and/or vomiting
- Yellow/brown discoloration of growing teeth
- Diarrhoea
- Skin rashes, including urticaria
- Hypersensitivity reactions: angioedema/anaphylaxis
- Benign intracranial hypertension.

Significant interactions

Tetracyclines are poorly absorbed in the gastrointestinal tract and their absorption is further impaired by antacids, including cows' milk, calcium, magnesium or aluminium salts.

Drugs that block bacterial metabolic pathways

Sulphonamides

Mechanism of action

These drugs are less commonly used now than in the past, as a result of the development of bacterial resistance. They are used in combination with other agents, especially trimethoprim, and can be extremely effective as a result of synergistic activity.

Both the sulphonamides and trimethoprim block the metabolic pathway of p-aminobenzoic acid (PABA), which is involved in the formation of para-purines and pyrimidines (Figure 11.2). The sulphonamides are PABA analogues, whereas trimethoprim acts as an inhibitor of dihydrofolate reductase.

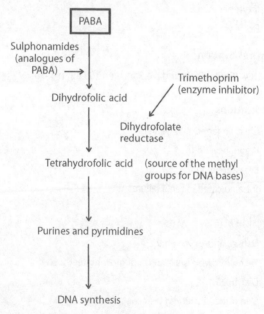

Figure 11.2 Metabolic pathway of para-aminobenzoic acid (PABA).

Example

Sulfamethoxazole.

Example prescription

CO-TRIMOXAZOLE 960 mg p.o. b.d.

This preparation contains a combination of trimethoprim and sulfamethoxazole in a ratio of 1:5.

Contraindication

Porphyria.

Common side effects

- Nausea and vomiting
- Hypersensitivity reactions, including erythema nodosum and the Stevens–Johnson syndrome
- Can cause kernicterus if given during the last trimester of pregnancy.

Significant interactions

- Risk of arrhythmia with amiodarone
- Increased anticoagulant effect of warfarin
- Increased risk of nephrotoxicity when given with ciclosporin.

Trimethoprim

Mechanism of action

This drug can be used alone or in combination with sulfamethoxazole (see above). It acts as an inhibitor of the enzyme dihydrofolate reductase, which blocks the synthesis of DNA.

Example prescription

TRIMETHOPRIM 200 mg p.o. b.d.

Contraindication

Blood dyscrasia.

Common side effects

- Nausea and/or vomiting
- Skin rashes
- Bone marrow suppression (caused by inhibition of folate metabolism).

Significant interactions

- Risk of arrhythmia with amiodarone
- Increased anticoagulant effect of warfarin
- Increased risk of nephrotoxicity when given with ciclosporin
- Increased phenytoin levels.

Drugs that prevent DNA or RNA replication

Quinolones

Mechanism of action

These drugs are bactericidal. They block the activity of the DNA gyrase enzyme, which is responsible for the formation of DNA supercoils. Without this function bacterial DNA cannot replicate or be repaired.

Examples

- Ciprofloxacin
- Ofloxacin
- Moxifloxacin.

Example prescription

CIPROFLOXACIN 500 mg p.o. b.d.

Contraindications

Moxifloxacin is not recommended in patients with a prolonged Q–T interval on the ECG or in people with liver impairment.

Common side effects

- Nausea, vomiting and/or diarrhoea
- Dizziness
- Skin rashes (especially photosensitivity rashes).

Significant interactions

- Moxifloxacin increases the risk of ventricular arrhythmias when combined with various types of drugs.
- Increased anticoagulant effect of warfarin.
- Increased risk of nephrotoxicity when given with ciclosporin.

Metronidazole

Mechanism of action

This drug is not itself bactericidal but must first be metabolised by the liver into an intermediate toxic metabolite, which not only inhibits DNA synthesis but also causes bacterial DNA to break down. Some species of bacteria and protozoal organisms are capable of metabolising metronidazole to its toxic metabolite. This means that it can also be used to treat some protozoal infections, eg *Giardia lamblia*.

The drug is well absorbed by mouth or across mucosal surfaces, which means that it can be given as an oral preparation or as vaginal or rectal suppositories.

Example prescription

METRONIDAZOLE 400 mg p.o. t.i.d.

Contraindication

Porphyria.

Common side effects

- Nausea
- Skin rashes
- Vomiting after alcohol (an effect similar to that of disulfiram) – patients should be warned not to drink alcohol while taking this drug.

Significant interactions

- Increased anticoagulant effect of warfarin
- Increased phenytoin levels.

Nitrofurantoin

Mechanism of action

Once this drug enters bacteria, it is converted to an unstable metabolite that damages bacterial DNA and results in cell death. This effect is maximal with *E. coli* in acid urine, and therefore this drug is used almost exclusively for urinary tract infections. As tissue concentrations are low, this antibiotic is not recommended for anything other than lower urinary tract infection.

Example prescription

NITROFURANTOIN 50 mg p.o. q.i.d.

Contraindications

- Porphyria
- Renal impairment
- Glucose-6-phosphate dehydrogenase deficiency.

Common side effects

- Nausea and vomiting
- Long-term use can cause pulmonary symptoms as a result of allergic pneumonitis.

Significant interactions

None.

Box 11.1 Antibiotics in common use

Penicillins	**Polymyxins**	**Tetracyclines**
Benzylpenicillin	Colistin	Tetracycline
Phenoxymethylpenicillin	**Vancomycin**	Oxytetracycline
Amoxicillin	**Macrolides**	Doxycycline
Ampicillin	Erythromycin	**Sulphonamides**
Co-amoxiclav	Clarithromycin	Sulfamethoxazole
Flucloxacillin	**Lincosamides**	**Trimethoprim**
Ticarcillin	Clindamycin	**Quinolones**
Piperacillin	**Aminoglycosides**	Ciprofloxacin
Cephalosporins	Gentamicin	**Metronidazole**
Cefalexin	Streptomycin	**Nitrofurantoin**
Cefuroxime	Tobramycin	
Cefotaxime	**Fusidic acid**	

Guidelines for antibiotic treatment regimens

For all of these diseases, it is essential, if possible, to establish the causative organism and antibiotic sensitivities. There are a number of options, but in all cases patients should be asked about antibiotic allergies/hypersensitivities and if these are present alternative antibiotics should be used (Table 11.1).

Table 11.1 Treatment regimens for bacterial infections

Tonsillitis and pharyngitis

Aetiology	*Streptococci*
Suggested treatment	AMOXICILLIN 250–500 mg p.o. or i.v. q.i.d., or
	CO-AMOXICLAV 625 mg p.o. t.i.d.
Alternatives	ERYTHROMYCIN 250–500 mg p.o. q.i.d., or
	CLARITHROMYCIN 250 mg p.o. b.d.

Quinsy

Aetiology	*Streptococci*
Suggested treatment	BENZYLPENICILLIN 1.2 g i.m. or i.v. 4-hourly
Alternative	CLARITHROMYCIN 500 mg i.v. b.d. then p.o. if able to swallow

Community-acquired pneumonia

Aetiology	*Pneumococci, H. influenzae, M. catarrhalis*
Suggested treatment	AMOXICILLIN 500 mg p.o. t.i.d., or
	AMPICILLIN 500 mg p.o. q.i.d., or
	CO-AMOXICLAV 625 mg p.o. t.i.d.
Alternative	CLARITHROMYCIN 500 mg p.o. b.d.

Infective exacerbation of chronic obstructive airway disease

Aetiology	*Pneumococci, H. influenzae, M. catarrhalis*
Suggested treatment	AMOXICILLIN 500 mg p.o. t.i.d., or
	CO-AMOXICLAV 1.2 g p.o. i.v. t.i.d. or 625 mg p.o. t.i.d.
Alternative	CLARITHROMYCIN 500 mg p.o. or i.v. b.d.

Hospital-acquired pneumonia

Aetiology	*Enterobacteria, S. aureus*
Suggested treatment	CEFOTAXIME 1 g i.v. t.i.d. ± GENTAMICIN
Alternative	CIPROFLOXACIN 500 mg p.o. b.d. or 400 mg i.v. b.d. +
	CLINDAMYCIN 600 mg i.v. q.i.d. ± GENTAMICIN

Aspiration pneumonia

Aetiology	Anaerobic bacteria, *streptococci*
Suggested treatment	CO-AMOXICLAV 1.2 g i.v. t.i.d.
Alternative	CLINDAMYCIN 600 mg i.v. q.i.d.

Table 11.1 Treatment regimens for bacterial infections *(continued)*

Lower urinary tract infection

Aetiology	*E. coli*, coagulase-negative *staphylococci*, *enterobacteria*
Suggested treatment	TRIMETHOPRIM 200 mg p.o. b.d., or CO-TRIMOXAZOLE 960 mg p.o. b.d., or NITROFURANTOIN 50 mg p.o. q.i.d.
Alternative	CEFALEXIN 250 mg p.o. q.i.d.

Pyelonephritis

Aetiology	*Enterobacteria, enterococci,* coagulase-negative *staphylococci*
Suggested treatment	CIPROFLOXACIN 500 mg p.o. b.d. or 400 mg i.v. b.d. ± GENTAMICIN 5 mg/kg i.v. o.d. (guided by peak and trough levels)

Cellulitis

Aetiology	Group A *streptococci, S. aureus*
Suggested treatment	FLUCLOXACILLIN 2 g i.v. q.i.d., and BENZYLPENCILLIN 1.2 g i.v. q.i.d.
Alternative	CLINDAMYCIN 600 mg i.v. q.i.d.

Abscesses

Aetiology	*Staphylococci, streptococci, Bacteroides*, enterobacteria
Suggested treatment	FLUCLOXACILLIN 500 mg i.v. q.i.d., or CEFUROXIME 1.5 g i.v. t.i.d., and METRONIDAZOLE 500 mg i.v. t.i.d.
Alternative	CLINDAMYCIN 600 mg i.v. q.i.d., and CIPROFLOXACIN 400 mg i.v. b.d.

Septicaemia

Aetiology	*Enterobacteria, staphylococci, streptococci*, others
Suggested treatment	PIPERACILLIN 4.5 g i.v. t.i.d., and GENTAMICIN 5 mg/kg i.v. o.d. (guided by peak and trough levels)
Alternative	CIPROFLOXACIN 400 mg i.v. b.d., and CLINDAMYCIN 600 mg i.v. q.i.d. ± GENTAMICIN 5 mg/kg i.v. o.d. (as above)

Bacterial meningitis

Aetiology	*Neisseria meningitidis, Streptococcus pneumoniae, H. influenzae*
Suggested treatment	CEFOTAXIME 2 g i.v. q.i.d.
Alternative	CHLORAMPHENICOL 25 mg/kg i.v. q.i.d.

Table 11.1 Treatment regimens for bacterial infections *(continued)*

Diabetic foot infection

Aetiology	Mixed organisms including anaerobes
Suggested treatment	CO-AMOXICLAV 1.2 g i.v. t.i.d., or
	FLUCLOXACILLIN 2 g i.v. q.i.d.
	± CIPROFLOXACIN 400 mg i.v. b.d.
	± METRONIDAZOLE 500 mg i.v. t.i.d.
Alternative	CLINDAMYCIN 600 mg i.v. q.i.d.
	+ CIPROFLOXACIN 400 mg i.v. b.d.

Septic arthritis

Aetiology	*S. aureus, streptococci*
Suggested treatment	FLUCLOXACILLIN 2 g i.v. q.i.d., and
	BENZYLPENCILLIN 1.2 g i.v. q.i.d.
Alternative	CLINDAMYCIN 600 mg i.v. q.i.d., and
	FUSIDIC ACID 500 mg i.v. t.i.d.

Wound infection

Aetiology	*S. aureus, streptococci*
Suggested treatment	FLUCLOXACILLIN 2 g i.v. q.i.d., and
	BENZYLPENICILLIN 1. 2 g i.v. q.i.d.
Alternative	CLINDAMYCIN 600 mg i.v. q.i.d.

Intra-abdominal abscess

Aetiology	*Enterobacteria*, anaerobes, *staphylococci, streptococci*
Suggested treatment	CEFUROXIME 1.5 g i.v. t.i.d., and
	METRONIDAZOLE 500 mg i.v. t.i.d.
Alternative	CLINDAMYCIN 600 mg i.v. q.i.d., and
	CIPROFLOXACIN 400 mg i.v. b.d.

Diverticulitis

Aetiology	*Enterobacteria*, anaerobes
Suggested treatment	CEFUROXIME 1.5 g i.v. t.i.d., and
	METRONIDAZOLE 500 mg i.v. t.i.d.
Alternative	CIPROFLOXACIN 400 mg i.v. b.d., and
	METRONIDAZOLE 500 mg i.v. t.i.d.

Cholecystitis

Aetiology	*Enterococci*, anaerobes, *enterobacteria*
Suggested treatment	AMPICILLIN 2 g i.v. q.i.d., and
	CIPROFLOXACIN 400 mg i.v. b.d.
Alternative	CLINDAMYCIN 600 mg i.v. q.i.d., and
	CIPROFLOXACIN 400 mg i.v. b.d.
	± GENTAMICIN 5 mg/kg i.v. o.d. (guided by peak and trough levels)

Table 11.1 Treatment regimens for bacterial infections *(continued)*

Tuberculosis (TB)

Aetiology	*Mycobacterium tuberculosis*
Suggested treatment	As a result of the risk of developing resistance to single antibiotics, TB is treated with a regimen of multiple drugs. Usually three drugs are used in combination for the first 2 months (until sensitivities have been determined), and then two drugs are used for a further 6 months.

For first 2 months

PYRAZINAMIDE 2.5 g p.o. three times per week

RIFAMPICIN 600–900 mg p.o. three times per week

ISONIAZID 15 mg/kg body weight p.o. three times per week

For months 3–6

RIFAMPICIN + ISONIAZID combination (Rifinah–300®) two tablets/day

In cases where organisms are shown to be resistant to isoniazid, ETHAMBUTOL 30 mg/kg can be used for the initial 2 months

Unwanted effects of anti-TB drugs

Isoniazid

Peripheral neuropathy

Hepatitis (uncommon)

Psychosis (rare)

Rifampicin

Liver damage

Influenza-like illness

Abdominal pain

Renal impairment

Thrombocytopenia

Liver enzyme induction, which may accelerate the metabolism of several drugs, including oestrogens (oral contraception pill), corticosteroids, phenytoin, sulphonylureas and anticoagulants

Pyrazinamide

Liver call damage (uncommon)

Ethambutol

Loss of visual acuity

Colour blindness

Restriction of visual fields

Antiviral drugs

The mode of action of antiviral drugs varies and is dependent to some extent on the type of virus targeted (DNA or RNA). These drugs can act at different points in the infection/replication pathway, which is shown in Figure 11.3.

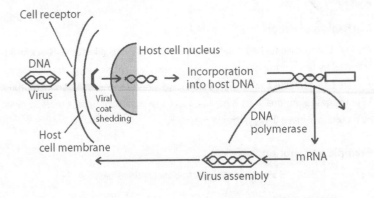

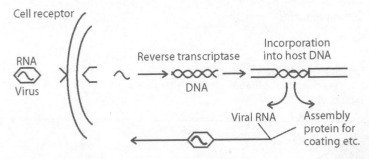

Figure 11.3 Infection with (a) DNA and (b) RNA viruses.

Viral DNA polymerase inhibitors

These drugs are active against DNA viruses. They inhibit the synthesis of viral DNA by acting as analogues for DNA bases. They affect only host cells that have virus particles present because they require phosphorylation by virus enzymes.

Aciclovir

Mechanism of action

Aciclovir is best used for herpes infections. Within DNA virus-infected cells, aciclovir is activated by being phosphorylated by the herpes virus enzyme thymidine kinase. The activated drug inhibits viral DNA polymerase, which stops viral replication. Absorption from the gastrointestinal tract is not good and so a significant dosage must be given by mouth to achieve therapeutic plasma levels.

Example prescriptions

ACICLOVIR 5% cream topically four to five times daily

ACICLOVIR 200 mg p.o. q.i.d.

Contraindications

None.

Common side effects

Topical

Few side effects.

Oral

- Nausea and/or vomiting
- Diarrhoea
- Urticaria/angioedema
- Itch
- Dizziness/confusion/drowsiness.

Intravenous

- Local inflammation of veins or thrombophlebitis
- Renal impairment
- Fever
- Psychosis
- Convulsions.

Significant interactions

None.

Ganciclovir

Mechanism of action

This drug is not activated by herpes virus enzymes, but by a different protein kinase enzyme that is present in cytomegalovirus (CMV). It is therefore the drug of choice for CMV infection. The drug is not absorbed when given by mouth and must be given by intravenous infusion.

Example prescription

> GANCICLOVIR 300 mg i.v. b.d.

Contraindications

- Pregnancy
- Breast-feeding
- Low blood cell counts.

Common side effects

- Thrombophlebitis
- Nausea
- Bone marrow suppression
- Skin rashes
- Encephalopathy
- Renal impairment
- Azoospermia in males.

Significant interactions

None.

RNA reverse transcriptase inhibitors

Mechanism of action

This group of drugs is active against the RNA viruses that rely on reverse transcriptase to become incorporated into the DNA of infected host cells. These drugs are activated within virally infected cells by phosphorylation. The activated drug inhibits the reverse transcriptase enzyme.

Examples

- Zidovudine
- Zalcitabine.

Example prescription

ZIDOVUDINE 250 mg p.o. t.i.d.

Contraindications

- Breast-feeding
- Low cell counts.

Common side effects

- Nausea and vomiting
- Oral ulceration
- Peripheral neuropathy
- Headache
- Pancreatitis
- Bone marrow suppression
- Liver cell damage
- Myalgia/myositis.

Significant interaction

Risk of myelosuppression when prescribed with ganciclovir.

RNA protease inhibitors

Mechanism of action

These drugs interfere with viral RNA protease enzymes and therefore affect the ability of a virus to produce polyproteins, which are required for viral replication. Production of the viral envelope is impaired for example.

Examples

- Saquinavir
- Indinavir.

Example prescription

> SAQUINAVIR 1 g p.o. b.d. within 2 hours of a meal

Contraindication

Breast-feeding.

Common side effects

- Nausea and vomiting
- Diarrhoea
- Liver cell damage
- Pancreatitis
- Bone marrow suppression
- Oral ulceration
- Headache
- Myalgia
- Peripheral neuropathy
- Renal stones.

Significant interactions

These drugs inhibit cytochrome P450 enzymes, and can therefore affect the action of other drugs that are metabolised by this enzyme system (see page 12).

Non-nucleoside analogue DNA polymerase inhibitors

Mechanism of action

These compounds bind to pyrophosphate binding sites on viral DNA polymerase, and prevent elongation of the DNA chain. They have an affinity that is approximately 100 times greater for viral DNA polymerase than for the human cell enzyme. They are used to treat herpes and CMV infections. These drugs can only be given by intravenous infusion because they are not absorbed when given by mouth.

Example

Foscarnet.

Example prescription

FOSCARNET 4.2 g i.v. t.i.d.

Contraindications

- Pregnancy
- Breast-feeding.

Common side effects

- Nausea, vomiting and/or diarrhoea
- Anorexia
- Abdominal pains
- Headache
- Paraesthesiae
- Renal toxicity
- Hypocalcaemia
- Liver cell damage
- Bone marrow suppression
- Thrombophlebitis.

Significant interactions

None.

Guidelines for antiviral treatment regimens (Box 11.2)

Box 11.2 Guidelines to antiviral treatment regimens

Herpes simplex

Oral lesions – topical aciclovir cream/ointment

Genital herpes – oral aciclovir for 5 days for acute lesions ± prophylactic therapy

Herpes zoster

Aciclovir given by mouth reduces the acute pain and post-herpetic neuralgia, if given at an early stage in the condition

+ analgesics

± gabapentin (see page 148)

Cytomegalovirus infection

Usually self-limiting but for patients with immunodeficiency or those with ocular infection or major organ involvement, ganciclovir intravenous infusions ± hyperimmune CMV immunoglobulin infusion.

Human immunodeficiency virus (HIV)

This virus infection is treated using a protease inhibitor drug together with two reverse transcriptase inhibitors:

Saquinavir

Zidovudine

Zalcitabine

If possible, treatment should be given before significant immunodeficiency has developed and if possible within 4–6 months of the seroconversion illness. If resistance occurs, two drugs should be changed. The aim of therapy is to reduce the viral load so that viral antigens cannot be found in the circulation.

Antifungal drugs

Most fungal infections occur on mucous membranes, in the skin or nails. Systemic fungal infections mainly affect patients with immunodeficiency disorders or individuals taking immunosuppressive drugs. The mechanisms of action of antifungal drugs are summarised in Figure 11.4.

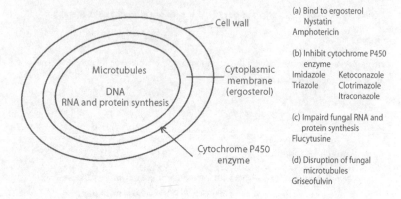

Figure 11.4 Modes of action of antifungal drugs.

Polyenes

Mechanism of action

These drugs bind to ergosterol in the cell wall of fungi and damage the active transport mechanism. Nystatin is not absorbed from the gastrointestinal tract, and amphotericin is only poorly absorbed. Both are used topically to treat skin and mucosal infections. Amphotericin can be given intravenously for systemic infections. It is excreted both by the kidneys and in bile, but very slowly, and therefore has an extremely long half-life of about 14 days. Both drugs can be used not only as an oral suspension but as topical creams, lozenges, ointments or pessaries.

Examples

- Nystatin
- Amphotericin.

Example prescription

> NYSTATIN oral suspension 100 000 units/ml – 1 ml p.o. q.i.d.

Contraindications

None.

Common side effects

Nystatin is an extremely safe drug and has virtually no side effects; intravenous amphotericin, on the other hand, can result in:

- Anorexia, nausea and/or vomiting
- Fever
- Renal impairment.

Significant interaction

Increased risk of nephrotoxicity when given with ciclosporin.

Imidazoles and triazoles

Mechanism of action

These drugs also act on the cell membrane of fungi and inhibit the cytochrome P450 enzyme 14α-demethylase, which is needed to convert lanosterol to ergosterol.

Imidazoles

Examples

- Ketoconazole
- Clotrimazole.

Example prescription

> KETOCONAZOLE 200 mg p.o. o.d.

Contraindications

- Liver impairment
- Pregnancy
- Breast-feeding.

Common side effects

- Nausea and vomiting
- Liver cell damage
- Gynaecomastia in males
- Oligospermia in males.

Significant interactions

This class of drug has multiple potential interactions. Always refer to the *BNF* interactions section before prescribing one of these agents.

Triazoles

Examples

- Itraconazole
- Fluconazole.

Example prescription

FLUCONAZOLE 150 mg p.o. o.d.

Contraindications

None.

Common side effects

- Nausea and vomiting
- Abdominal pain
- Diarrhoea
- Disturbance of liver function
- Stevens–Johnson syndrome
- Dizziness
- Seizures
- Headache
- Bone marrow suppression
- Alopecia
- Hypokalaemia.

Significant interactions

This class of drug has multiple potential interactions. Always refer to the *BNF* interactions section before prescribing one of these agents.

Flucytosine

Mechanism of action

This drug is converted to 5-fluorouracil by fungi. This then acts as an antimetabolite by competing with uracil for incorporation into the RNA of the fungus.

Example prescription

FLUCYTOSINE 3 g i.v. q.i.d.

Contraindications

None.

Common side effects

- Nausea and vomiting
- Diarrhoea
- Skin rashes
- Confusion/hallucinations
- Headache
- Convulsions
- Disturbance of liver function
- Bone marrow suppression.

Significant interactions

None.

Griseofulvin

Mechanism of action

This drug acts by inhibiting microtubule protein polymerisation of skin fungi and is therefore used to treat skin, scalp, hair and nail infections.

Example prescription

> GRISEOFULVIN 500 mg p.o. o.d.

Contraindications

- Liver disease
- Systemic lupus erythematosus (SLE)
- Porphyria
- Pregnancy
- Breast-feeding
- Men who wish to father a child in the 6 months after treatment.

Common side effects

- Nausea and vomiting
- Headache
- Photosensitivity
- Erythema multiforme
- Peripheral neuropathy
- Confusion
- Impaired coordination
- SLE.

Significant interactions

- Reduces the anticoagulant effect of warfarin
- Increases the metabolism of oestrogen and progestogens (reduces contraceptive effects)
- Increases the effects of alcohol.

Guidelines for antifungal treatment regimens

For guidelines see Box 11.3.

Box 11.3 Guidelines to antifungal treatment regimens

Oral candida infection

NYSTATIN oral suspension (100 000 units/ml) 1 ml held in mouth q.i.d., or

NYSTATIN pastilles one p.o. after each meal, or

AMPHOTERICIN lozenges one p.o. q.i.d.

Genital candidal infection

NYSTATIN cream 4 g topical b.d. for 14 days, and

NYSTATIN vaginal pessaries one or two inserted at night, or

CLOTRIMAZOLE 1% cream topical b.d. or t.i.d. for 6 days, and

CLOTRIMAZOLE pessaries one or two inserted at night for 6 nights

Tinea pedis (athlete's foot)

NYSTATIN cream or ointment topical b.d. or t.i.d., or

MICONAZOLE powder or cream topical b.d.

Fungal skin/scalp infection

NYSTATIN cream or ointment topical b.d. or t.i.d., or

MICONAZOLE cream topical b.d.

Onychomycosis (fungal nail infection)

GRISEOFULVIN 250mg p.o. b.d.

Systemic fungal infections

KETOCONAZOLE 200mg p.o. o.d. for 14 days, or

AMPHOTERICIN infusion ± FLUCYTOSINE, or

ITRACONAZOLE infusion

For dosage of infusion see individual product literature.

Antiparasitic drugs

Prophylaxis against malaria

Drugs are given to travellers before, during and after their visits to endemic areas. The type of prophylactic drug used depends on the region to be visited. If drug resistance is low, chloroquine or proguanil can be used; for areas where resistance is more of a problem, both drugs are used in combination; and in areas where chloroquine resistance is high, mefloquine is used.

Low risk of chloroquine resistance

CHLOROQUINE 300 mg p.o. once per week for 1–2 weeks before travelling, during stay and for 4 weeks after leaving endemic area, or

PROGUANIL 200 mg p.o. o.d. 1–2 weeks before travelling, during stay and for 4 weeks after leaving endemic area

Significant risk of chloroquine resistance

CHLOROQUINE 250 mg p.o. once per week, and

PROGUANIL 100 mg p.o. o.d. for 1–2 weeks before, during and 4 weeks after leaving endemic area

High risk of chloroquine resistance

MEFLOQUINE 250 mg p.o. once per week for 2–3 weeks before travelling, during stay and for 4 weeks after leaving endemic area

Treatment of malaria

Chloroquine

Mechanism of action

Chloroquine becomes concentrated within red cells that contain the malarial parasites because it binds avidly to a breakdown product of haemoglobin. The levels of chloroquine within infected red cells are approximately 100 times those found in the plasma. Within the red cells, the drug alters the pH of lysosomes, prevents haemoglobin degradation and may inhibit DNA and RNA function of the parasites. It is also concentrated in tissues containing melanin, for example liver, spleen, kidney and retina. Chloroquine has a long half-life (about 6 days) and therefore a once-per-week dosage schedule is adequate to maintain blood and tissue levels.

Chloroquine is used in the treatment of *Plasmodium vivax, malariae* or *ovale* malaria. It is not recommended for the treatment of *Plasmpodium falciparum* malaria.

Example prescription

CHLOROQUINE 600 mg p.o. stat, then 300 mg after 6–8 hours, followed by 300 mg o.d. for 2 days

Contraindications

None.

Common side effects

- Nausea, vomiting and/or diarrhoea
- Retinopathy (pigmentation), impaired visual activity and/or visual field defects
- Skin rashes.

Significant interactions

- Risk of arrhythmia when given with amiodarone or moxifloxacin
- Risk of ciclosporin toxicity.

Quinine

Mechanism of action

Quinine's antimalarial action is similar to that of chloroquine, although it does not bind to parasitic DNA. The drug can be used for all forms of malaria. For *P. falciparum* malaria, it is often used in combination with mefloquine (see below).

Example prescription

QUININE 600 mg p.o. t.i.d. for 7 days

Contraindications

- Myasthenia gravis
- Optic neuritis
- Haemoglobinuria.

Common side effects

- Nausea and vomiting
- Tinnitus and/or vertigo
- Headache
- Bradycardia
- Heart block
- Hearing loss.

Significant interactions

- Risk of arrhythmia when prescribed with certain antipsychotics, for example thioridazine
- Increased plasma levels of digoxin.

Mefloquine

Mechanism of action

This drug has a similar mode of action to chloroquine and quinine, but like quinine does not bind on to parasitic DNA. It is often used with quinine in the setting of chloroquine resistance. Mefloquine has a long half-life (about 3 weeks), meaning that a single dose gives adequate therapeutic drug levels for 3–4 weeks.

Example prescription

MEFLOQUINE 1.2 g p.o. as a single dose

Contraindications

- Neuropsychiatric disorders
- Convulsions
- Hypersensitivity to quinine.

Common side effects

- Nausea and vomiting
- Headache
- Vertigo
- Depression
- Psychosis, especially in patients with a previous psychiatric history.

Significant interactions

- Risk of arrhythmia when given with amiodarone, moxifloxacin or the antipsychotic pimozide
- Reduced action of anticonvulsants.

Treatment of *Pneumocystis carinii*

Co-trimoxazole

This drug is the drug of choice for *Pneumocystis carinii* infection but must be given at high dosage. See page 260 for more details.

Pentamidine

Mechanism of action

This drug is used for a number of protozoal infections, including *P. carinii*, trypanosomiasis and leishmaniasis. The drug is actively taken up by the protozoal organism, in which it inhibits protein synthesis in ribosomes. This results in the death of the organism. The drug is administered by intravenous injection or nebulised inhalation.

Example prescription

> PENTAMIDINE 280 mg i.v. o.d. for 14 days

Contraindications

None.

Common side effects

Intravenous

- Hypotension
- Renal impairment
- Hypoglycaemia
- Cardiac arrhythmias, including ventricular tachycardia.

Inhaled

Cough and/or bronchospasm.

Significant interactions

Risk of ventricular arrhythmias when given with amiodarone, moxifloxacin, terfenadine, amisulpride or thioridazine.

Treatment of *Giardia lamblia*

This protozoal infection is treated by giving oral metronidazole at a dose of 400 mg p.o. t.i.d. for 5 days (see page 263 for further details).

Treatment of toxoplasmosis

Most cases are self-limiting, but drug treatment is required if eye involvement or brain infection occurs, and in patients with immunodeficiency.

Pyrimethamine

Mechanism of action

This drug is a folate antagonist, and acts by inhibiting the enzyme dihydrofolate reductase. It should be used together with sulfadiazine (see below).

Contraindication

Porphyria.

Common side effects

- Mouth ulcers
- Dyspepsia.

Significant interactions

- Anti-folate effect increased with sulphonamides, trimethoprim, phenytoin, proguanil and methotrexate
- Reduced effect of phenytoin.

Sulfadiazine

This is a sulphonamide and has a similar mechanism of action and side-effect profile as sulfamethoxazole (see page 260). It can be given orally or by intravenous infusion and is used in combination with pyrimethamine to treat the serious complications of toxoplasmosis.

Treatment of amoebiasis

This protozoal infection is treated with metronidazole at a dose of 800 mg p.o. t.i.d. for 5 days (see page 263 for details).

Treatment of helminth infections

Benzimidazoles

Mechanism of action

A variety of helminths, including threadworms, roundworms, tapeworms and hookworms, can infect humans. Benzimidazoles act by specifically binding to parasite tubulin, and preventing it from forming the cytoskeleton of the microtubules. They damage not only the adult worms but also the larvae. Mebendazole is poorly absorbed from the gut and therefore high levels are available to be taken up by the parasites.

Example prescription

> MEBENDAZOLE 100 mg p.o. stat

Contraindication

Pregnancy.

Common side effects

- Diarrhoea
- Abdominal pain
- Skin rashes.

Significant interactions

None.

12
Poisoning

Management of the poisoned patient
Paracetamol overdose

12
Poisoning

Management of the poisoned patient

This chapter details the general management of a patient who has been poisoned. Specific details on the management of paracetamol poisoning are given at the end of the chapter.

Supportive care, ie keeping the patient alive while the body excretes or metabolises the drug naturally, is generally the most important part of managing a poisoned patient. In certain circumstances, antidotes may be necessary, and other modalities are occasionally used to clear drugs more quickly from the body.

General measures

If the patient is unconscious, treat as for any emergency using the **ABCDE** approach.

Airway

The airway should be cleared, and maintained if necessary with airway adjuncts such as an oropharyngeal or nasopharyngeal airway. A laryngeal mask airway or endotracheal tube may be required in certain circumstances. Oxygen should be administered.

Breathing

A rapid assessment of respiration rate and auscultation of the lungs should be carried out. Haemoglobin saturation should be measured using a finger probe. If respiratory effort is suboptimal, ventilatory support may be required. This may involve augmenting the patient's breathing using a bag-valve-mask system, or connection to a ventilator.

Circulation

The pulse, blood pressure and capillary refill time should be assessed. A cardiac monitor should be attached. Intravenous access must be obtained and fluids administered as appropriate to ensure adequate perfusion.

Disability

Never forget to check the capillary blood glucose level in an unconscious patient. If hypoglycaemia is confirmed, give 50 ml 50% dextrose intravenously, followed by a copious flush (eg 50 ml 0.9% saline).

Next assess the level of consciousness (eg using the AVPU system or Glasgow Coma Scale [GCS] – Box 12.1), and inspect the pupils for asymmetry and reactivity to light. Abnormalities may point to intracranial pathology, eg a patient who has collapsed and sustained a head injury after a drug overdose may develop an extradural haematoma, which should be suspected in the setting of a unilateral fixed and dilated pupil.

Exposure

Perform a complete head-to-toe examination of the patient to ensure that you are not missing something.

In addition:

- Treat seizures with LORAZEPAM 2–4 mg i.v.. Intravenous or rectal DIAZEPAM is an alternative.
- If there is any reason to suspect opiate toxicity (eg respiratory rate less than 12/minute or pinpoint pupils), give NALOXONE.
- Unless unconscious, nurse the patient semi-prone (to prevent inhalation of gastric contents).
- Rewarm if hypothermic.

History

Ascertain what was taken, in what quantity and at what time. A brief psychiatric assessment should be carried out to investigate the reason for the overdose, the circumstances surrounding it and suicidal ideation.

All patients who have taken an overdose should be assessed by a psychiatrist during their admission.

Box 12.1 Assessing level of consciousness

AVPU system

Assess the patient as A, V, P or U depending on whether they are:

Alert
responding to Voice
responding to Pain
Unresponsive

Glasgow Coma Scale

Assess the patient according to the following three criteria and give them a total score of between 3 and 15:

Eyes

Open spontaneously	4
Open to voice	3
Open to pain	2
Do not open	1

Motor

Obeys commands	6
Localises pain	5
Withdraws to pain	4
Abnormal flexion to pain	3
Abnormal extension to pain	2
No response to pain	1

Voice

Orientated	5
Confused	4
Inappropriate words	3
Incomprehensible words	2
No speech	1

Reduce absorption of the poison

It would seem logical to try to reduce the amount of a drug that enters the bloodstream. However, there is very little evidence that any of the measures taken to reduce absorption actually affect morbidity or mortality. Methods employed include the following.

Decontamination

This would be applicable if a patient has been in *contact* with a toxic substance, rather than after drug ingestion. Options available include irrigation of the eyes, removal of contaminated clothing and thorough washing of the skin.

Gastric lavage

This should be considered if a patient presents to hospital within 1 hour of ingestion of a dangerous dose of a poison (4 hours if aspirin/salicylate has been taken). The airway must be protected if the patient has a reduced level of consciousness. Gastric lavage should *not* be performed if corrosives have been ingested or if there is any suspicion of oesophageal or gastric pathology.

Activated charcoal

Consider giving activated charcoal if a significant amount of a poison has been ingested, and the patient presents within 1 hour. Again, protect the airway if the patient is not fully conscious.

Please note that induced emesis and treatment with laxatives have no role to play in the management of a poisoned patient.

Enhance elimination of the poison

In certain circumstances, efforts can be made to speed up elimination of a poison from the body. Options available include those summarised opposite.

Repeated dosing of activated charcoal

As noted above, a single dose of charcoal can reduce the absorption of a poison. In certain circumstances, multiple doses of activated charcoal are administered (eg 50 g every 4 hours) in order to enhance drug elimination. Charcoal has the ability to adsorb certain drugs, and it also interferes with the enterohepatic circulation. Repeated dosing of activated charcoal may be considered after overdosage of carbamazepine, dapsone, phenobarbital, quinine or theophylline.

Urinary alkalinisation

This technique makes use of the Henderson–Hasselbalch equation (see Chapter 1). Briefly, the pH of an environment determines whether a drug exists in an ionised or unionised form. In the renal tubules, only the unionised form of a drug will be reabsorbed. The idea here is therefore to change the pH of the urine in order to ionise the drug further, and therefore reduce resorption. More drug will then be excreted. Making the urine alkaline by administering sodium bicarbonate will increase the elimination of, for example, salicylates.

Dialysis (peritoneal or haemodialysis)

In the same manner as dialysis is used to clear toxins from the bodies of patients with renal failure, dialysis can be used to remove poisons after a drug overdose. The technique is suitable only for certain poisons, eg salicylates, phenobarbital, methanol, ethylene glycol and lithium.

Specific antidotes

Several important antidotes are available; the most commonly used are listed in Table 12.1. Always consider using an antidote when faced with a poisoned patient.

The Poisons Information Centres can always be consulted for guidance on treating poisoned patients.

Poison/overdose	Antidote
Anticholinergic agents	Physostigmine
Arsenic	Dimercaprol
Benzodiazepines	Flumazenil
Beta blockers	Glucagon
Calcium channel antagonists	Calcium gluconate
Carbon monoxide	Oxygen
Cyanide	Amyl nitrite, sodium nitrite, sodium thiosulphate, dicobalt edetate, hydroxycobalamin
Digoxin	Digoxin-specific antibody fragments
Ethylene glycol	Ethanol
Iron	Desferrioxamine
Lead	Dimercaprol or penicillamine
Mercury	Dimercaprol or penicillamine
Nitrates/nitrites	Methylthioninium chloride
Opiates	Naloxone*
Organophosphates	Atropine
Paracetamol	N-acetylcysteine or methionine
Paraquat	Fuller's earth
Phenothiazines	Benzatropine
Warfarin	Vitamin K or fresh frozen plasma

*Note: the half-life of naloxone is shorter than the half-life of most opiates. Therefore there is a tendency for this drug to wear off before the opiate itself. The patient may then exhibit features of opiate toxicity again, including respiratory depression. Always monitor such patients carefully. Further doses of naloxone may be necessary. Sometimes a naloxone infusion is required.

Table 12.1 Important antidotes

Paracetamol overdose

This is one of the most common forms of deliberate self-harm and often presents as an overdose of drug associated with excess alcohol intake or as ingestion with other drugs. Occasionally patients are seen who accidentally overdose because of frequent analgesic use in an attempt to obtain pain relief. Serious liver damage can occur with as few as 15 x 500 mg tablets taken in a 24-hour period.

Paracetamol is normally metabolised in the liver by conjugation to harmless glucuronide or sulphate conjugates, with a small amount being oxidised by the cytochrome P450 system to a reactive metabolite (N-Acetyl-p-benzoquinoneimine). This metabolite is conjugated with thiol groups from glutathione, resulting in its inactivation. In significant overdose, the normal conjugation pathways are saturated. High levels of N-acetyl-p-benzoquinoneimine accumulate within liver cells and deplete glutathione stores. The reactive metabolite is then free to form covalent bonds with intracellular macromolecules and cause cell necrosis (Figure 12.1).

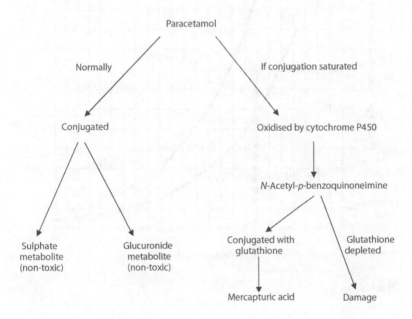

Figure 12.1 Metabolism of paracetamol.

Administration of the antidote N-acetylcysteine (NAC) aims to augment liver stores of glutathione, and thus reduce or prevent liver damage. However, NAC administration is not without its problems, eg there is a risk of anaphylaxis. It is therefore not routinely given to all patients who have taken paracetamol in excess. To decide who should receive NAC, the nomogram in Figure 12.2 should be used.

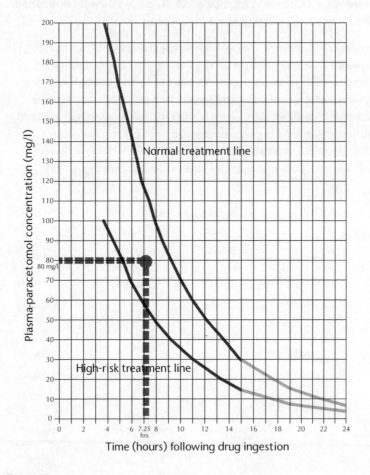

Figure 12.2

It is critical to know when the paracetamol was taken, and to measure the blood level 4 hours after this time. In suspected major overdoses (> 12 g), NAC may be given presumptively on presentation, but blood levels should always be checked at 4 hours.

Note the two lines on the graph in Figure 12.2. In routine circumstances, use the normal treatment line. Plot the blood concentration of paracetamol against the time after ingestion and compare this point with the treatment line. If it is on or above the line, treatment should be given. If it is below, there is no indication for treatment. Some patients are deemed 'high risk' for liver damage (see Box 12.2), and for them the 'high-risk treatment line' should be used. Such patients are presumed to have lower than normal antioxidant stores.

Box 12.2 Patients at high risk in paracetamol overdose

Patients prescribed hepatic enzyme-inducing drugs (eg phenytoin, rifampicin, carbamazepine)

People with alcohol dependence

Malnourished people (including anorexia nervosa)

AIDS patients

Patients with chronic liver disease

Index

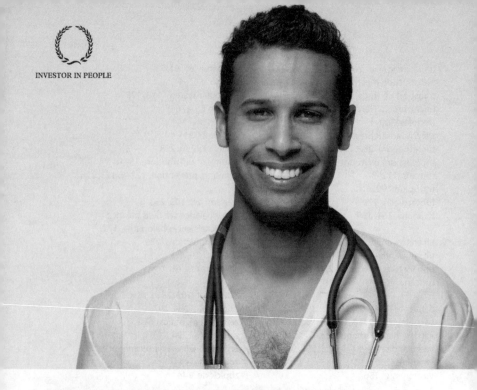

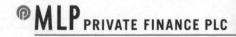